FIRST EDITION

Book cover design by Stacey Lane, Stacey Lane Design LLC, Denver, Colorado

Edited by Charol Messenger, Denver, Colorado

Library of Congress Cataloging-in-Publication Data:

Simendinger, Theodore J.
   How to Manage the Worry Circle/Theodore J. Simendinger as "Ocean Palmer." 1st edition.

ISBN: 978-0-9765485-3-9

1. Non-fiction   2. Self-help   3. Business
4. Professional Development   5. Title

Library of Congress Control Number: on file, case number 1-148911961

10 9 8 7 6 5 4 3 2 1

Published by Airplane Reader Publishing Company, Denver, Colorado U.S.A.

Printed in the United States of America

HOW TO MANAGE THE

WORRY CIRCLE

Manage The Circle!

by Ocean Palmer

DEDICATION

"I worry so much, I wonder what kind of wine goes with finger-nails."

—Milton Berle, comedian

It takes a team to create a good published work and I'm lucky to have a talented one. Featured are illustrator Stacey Lane, editor Charol Messenger, my good friend Chip Ford, and my brother Mark. Writing this book was an inspiring project, due largely to its simple, uncluttered motivation: to help people. I am also grateful to all the wonderful people I've met and worked with, across the globe and throughout the years. Together we've shared thousands of hours discussing what they worry about and why. Especially inspiring are those who better manage their Worry Circles. They are living a quote by Henry David Thoreau, written 150 years ago.

"Times do not change," he wrote. "We change."

But in many ways, the times *have* changed. The loud thunderclaps and crackling lightning bolts that menace from an uneasy economic storm will eventually give way to the next generation of bright, sunny days. Until they do, it's good to reminisce with another quote, this one by Dale Carnegie (back when $1 was worth today's $10).

"If only the people who worry about their liabilities would think about the riches they do possess, they would stop worrying. Would you sell both your eyes for a million dollars ... or your two legs ... or your hands ... or your hearing? Add up what you do have, and you'll find that you won't sell them for all the gold in the world. The best things in life are yours, if you can appreciate yourself."

Words to live by, for sure.

Table of Contents

How to Manage the Worry Circle

by Ocean Palmer

Chapter		Page
	Foreword	
1	Say Hello to Your Worry Circle	1
2	Lemme Guess Whatcha Got in Your Circle!	15
3	Self-caused Worries	21
4	Familial Worries	31
5	Social Worries	43
6	Environmental Worries	51
7	Work Worries	57
8	Money Worries	71
9	Varying Degrees of Worry Intensity	75
10	If Worries Are Invisible, Why Are They So Heavy?	81
11	Changing the Way You Keep Score	87
12	How to Manage The Worry Circle	91
13	Tips to Help Over the Long Haul	99
14	Crafting Your Daily Dozen	107
	Worksheet: Emptying Your Worry Circle	115

THE GREATEST GOLF SHOT I EVER SAW

I've never been a good golfer, but I've been lucky enough to watch the greats play. Technology has made it easier than ever for good players to hit super shots, but the most memorable ones I've seen were struck years ago.

In 1979, I watched tour star Lanny Wadkins win the Tournament Players Championship at Sawgrass Country Club by five shots over Tom Watson. The March winds howled so strongly that it was hard to wear a hat much less play golf. Yet time and again, Wadkins pounded fairway drivers straight and true on a course that seemed unplayable to mere mortals. Anybody can hit a driver off a tee, but very few can hit one accurately "off the deck." Wadkins was a master.

As great as Wadkins' talent was, the previous year on the same course, during Wednesday's practice round, Jack Nicklaus hit a shot I've never forgotten. His caddy back then was the frizzy-haired Angelo Argea. As usual, the Sawgrass wind was blowing like a baby tornado. I was standing by the green on a long par-five. From way back down the fairway, a flash of sparkling sunshine reflected off a steel shaft like a mirror. The recognizable swing belonged to Nicklaus. The golf ball was a speck, hurtling like a bullet, boring through the crosswind to a small green as hard as linoleum. The ball bounced on the front of the green, took a couple of hops and rolled toward the stick. It stopped pin-high, twelve feet right.

Caddy Argea, who had left the boss behind and gone ahead, walked over to repair the ball mark. Then he stood nearby to wait. I looked at him and asked, "How far?"

"252," he said. "One-iron."

I shook my head. "Nobody can do that."

Argea shrugged. "He can."

Hall of Famer Lee Trevino, who had won six majors and twenty-nine PGA tour events, used to regale that during lightning storms he always held a one-iron over his head, "Because even God can't hit a one-iron." Then he'd laugh.

For more than a decade, Jack Nicklaus' practice-round one-iron remained the greatest shot I ever saw. That changed after the PGA Tour opened its proud baby, Ponte Vedra's TPC at Sawgrass Stadium Course. The first few years, the course was grossly unfair. Hills and valleys created putting locations that were impossible, even for the greatest players in the world. The famed par-three island hole, number 17, wasn't the problem; it was putting a six-footer from above the hole on the eighth. You had to nudge the ball to get it started downhill, then sprint. The ball rolled and rolled and rolled and never stopped. I hit one a bit too firm once on a Monday that didn't stop rolling until Tuesday. My pal went next and fared even worse. His didn't quit rolling until the city limits of St. Augustine.

Even so, I loved that original, unfair layout. The greatest shot I ever saw came there, five minutes after I hit three straight career shots and tapped in a par putt on 18 for my TPC lifetime-best: 100. My buddy and I always played the course "from the tips," the pro tee boxes way back where the big boys played. Considering that I stank, it wasn't a good strategy.

Anyhow, after finishing our round, my buddy and I climbed back into our golf cart and wound our way back up toward the clubhouse, which back then was perched atop a high hill overlooking the sprawling campus. Near the top, my buddy suddenly jammed on the brakes. He'd noticed something down off in the distance to his left.

"C'mon," he urged. He climbed out of the cart and circled back to his golf bag.

I was puzzled but I got out and walked around to see what he was doing.

He pointed. "Down there. See him?"

The "him" was a bull gator, fourteen-feet long if he was an inch. The massive creature was sunning on the grassy bank of a retention pond. He was sound asleep and minding his own business. Dreaming of lady gators, no doubt.

"See him," I concurred. "So what?"

My pal pulled a wedge out of his bag. "I'm takin' a shot."

He walked to the front of the cart, found a flat spot, and threw down a ball. He gripped his wedge, measured the shot, glanced at the trees for a hint on the wind, and took dead aim.

I wasn't particularly concerned, since hitting a gator from ninety yards from the crest of a hill three stories up is about as easy as hitting a 252-yard one-iron pin-high in a howling crosswind.

My buddy's smooth swing whooshed through the grass. *"Pffft!"* The ball soared high, real high, straight and true toward where he aimed.

"It's on line," I muttered, wondering how close it might land to the target so far away. "Is it far enough?"

"Yep," he said. "It's close."

We stood there mesmerized by the ball in flight.

THUMP!

That golf ball landed dead-square on top of that gator's head, right between the eyes. In a blink, those eyes went from peacefully closed to angry wide. The ball rebounded ten feet high, which tells you how hard that bull gator's head was.

Gator hunters say it's the young ones you've got to watch out for, that the old ones don't move so fast. That's a lie. Conk one in the head with a Titleist from a hilltop ninety yards away and I guarantee you this: a big, angry gator can fly. That gator went from zero to sixty in a flash. Dove in, across, and back out of that retention pond and raced straight up the hill right for us.

We just stood and stared, frozen, expecting him to stop but he kept coming. His legs churned so fast they blurred like he was running on a dozen of them.

My buddy and I looked at each other, not sure what to do.

"He's ticked off!" I yelled, racing to my side of the golf cart.

"Let's get outta here!"

My buddy jumped aboard, too, still holding his wedge, and buried the accelerator. We lurched forward. If that gator was going to get us, he'd have to navigate the pro shop, climb down two flights of stairs, and corner us in the men's locker room.

That gator wedge shot remains the greatest I ever saw. Better than the holes-in-ones, better than the guy who buried a rented Chrysler New Yorker in a sand trap trying to park at the U.S. Open, even better than Tiger being Tiger.

My buddy who hit that shot, Dick Haase, is in a bit of medical stew right now. It's in his honor that I've written this book. Dick first broached the idea of the Worry Circle twenty years ago when we were playing golf in Ocala, hacking through the weeds. We talked about it, my research deepened, and I began teaching what you are about to read. This work has helped thousands of people across four continents all around the world and I'm very proud of that. I'm even prouder to be his friend.

Denver, Colorado

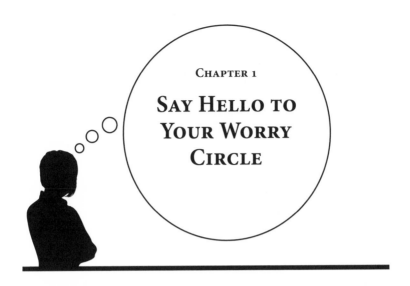

CHAPTER 1

SAY HELLO TO YOUR WORRY CIRCLE

What the heck is a Worry Circle? Hint: Everybody's got one.

The Worry Circle is an imaginary bubble each of us has where we carry all the things we worry about, fears and concerns of all kinds: personal, familial, social, environmental, professional, financial—anything and everything over which we stress.

Whether an issue is large or small, fleeting or long-lasting, it lives inside this Circle. To illustrate the Worry Circle in action, let's grab an imaginary flashlight and crawl inside your mind.

Following is a simple exercise. Take a minute to complete the top portion, Step #1. After you finish, resume reading. A few pages further, we'll return to Step #2.

"THE WORRY CIRCLE" ©

Focus on yourself for a few minutes!
(This is a personal exercise.)

Exercise 1

Inside the large circle, list all the things you worry about. If you run out of room, jot topics outside the circle, too. This is a chance to "purge," so take full advantage. Describe the obvious, but also carefully identify the not so obvious. After you have emptied your head of all the things you worry about, read on. We will come back to Exercise #2.

Exercise 2

Based on the instructions you're given to complete step #2, finish the exercise.

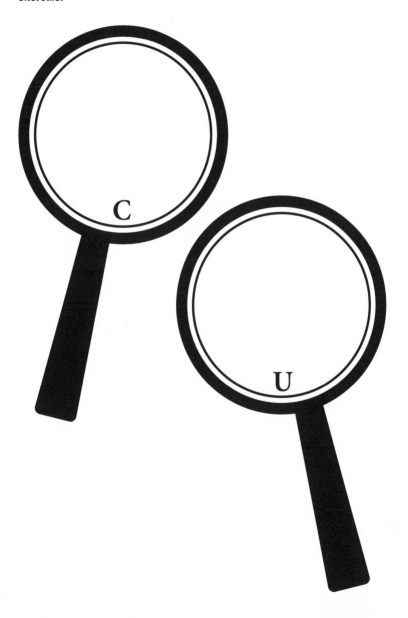

The Four Principles of the Worry Circle

In a tumbling economy, it's safe to assume that, for many, the Worry Circle is more crowded than ever. People are, by nature, herd animals, with a herd social structure and mentality. Change—real or imagined, anticipated or unexpected—is a common catalyst for worry. Change (or the threat of change) disrupts our status quo. Whenever change is thrust upon us, like the economy just did, we must adjust or adapt. When forced to adjust, the comfortable interconnections of our life are disrupted. Disruptions are stressful, so we worry. We are used to, and comfortable with, the way things have been, and we're uneasy until we've adjusted to the new rules of the new game.

The fundamental basis of the Worry Circle is accepting that worrying about "stuff" is a normal part of life. We recognize that worries will always exist in some form and degree. Life brings issues on a continuous escalator. Despite these things appearing in steady succession, we don't fear their arrival. Worry Circle management enables us to meet what we worry about head-on, and with confidence.

Here are the four guiding principles:

1. Worry is normal. Everyone does it. It's human nature.
2. The need to worry is relentless, but what we worry about comes and goes.
3. We worry about three kinds of things:
    - What we can control.
    - What we can influence but not control.

- What we can neither influence nor control.
4. There is a right way and a wrong way to deal with worry.

Although worry is inborn and seems endless, what we worry about changes all the time. When the roof leaks, we worry about the roof. Car problem, we worry about the car. The phone rings and our child has been injured, we forget about the roof and the car and panic over our child.

Worries come and go. When one worry is resolved, another slips into its place. They replace each other. Regardless of what fills our Worry Circle, our need to worry remains relentless. Life does not allow an empty Worry Circle.

What we worry about varies wildly and we all dwell on worries differently, largely due to the influences of our upbringing and personality. Some people have a low tolerance for worry and stress; others can sustain more weight. People with an expressive, outgoing "Type A" personality often seem to thrive on an ongoing chain of stressful events.

Reactive chaos seemed good in a thriving economy; it's not so good in a declining economy. The number, scope, and magnitude of today's worries are off the charts from what's familiar to us.

To a large extent, what people worry about is a choice. To choose wisely, we must learn what to think about and what not to think about … and we really do have a choice.

This workbook teaches what we should worry about and what we shouldn't worry about. It also shares how best to manage those choices with efficiency and confidence.

Three things typically determine how immersed we get in our worries:

- Our upbringing and core beliefs.
- Significant emotional events we've weathered.
- The amount of free time we have.

Most people are shaped into who they will be as adults based upon the blend of environmental factors that existed during their formative years. Such collective influences shape our "core beliefs," what we hold to be true about the world.

After our formative years, what changes us are significant emotional events, the impactful situations in life that alter our views and behaviors. These experiences can be good or bad, expected or unexpected. Face it, stuff happens. Because it happens, there's no such thing as "victimization." We embrace significant emotional events as inevitable and own the need to process these things, for better or worse, the best we can.

Like it or not, ready or not, we all have major emotional events thrust upon us. When they arrive, we don't fear them. We deal with them head-on, we do not retreat. How we react reshapes who we are becoming.

People who stay busy have less idle time to reflect; they also tend to have less time to worry. Worriers have plenty of time to stew. Busy people plan to worry later, if they have the time.

The blend of these three things—core beliefs, significant emotional events, and free time—has a major influence over how deeply we get immersed in our worries.

The Three Kinds of Worries

Things We Can Control

The only thing in life we can control is our thoughts, feelings, and behaviors. Being able to control a Worry Circle issue means we can remedy a concern by our behaviors. When we can address or retire a worry issue by our actions, it's a controllable issue. If our actions cannot fix an issue, it's uncontrollable.

Based on research, 62 percent of what people worry about falls into the controllable category, 38 percent does not. Since roughly three out of five things we worry about can be remedied by our personal actions, we must learn to accurately identify what we should or should not worry about.

Smart Worry Circle practitioners embrace policing their thoughts so they are concerned only with issues they can resolve by their behaviors. They waste no time or energy fretting over unsolvable problems.

Worrying about things we can control is a position of strength. When something controllable bugs us, we can deal with it.

Training our mind to worry only about things we can control is the crux of effective Worry Circle management. Specific techniques to manage controllable issues are in chapter twelve, including how to block out those 38 percent of things we typically worry about that we cannot control.

Things We Can Influence (but not control)

A worry we can influence features some portion we can

control but a resolution that is beyond our ability to solve. We may contribute a part of the solution. For example, we can be nice to others but not control what they think of us. We can be our best at work but not control the spaceman from another planet who writes a cockeyed performance appraisal. We can interview for a job that perfectly matches our talents but we can't control who gets the job.

Parenting falls heavily into the influence category. Moms and dads want to be good parents, but where does parental accountability end? Once our children start attending school, they are on their own to act as they decide. Often they do what their peers goad them into doing, sometimes even breaking the law. Away from parental guidance, children make choices, hopefully good choices. Most do, some don't.

What part of worrying should the parent own? Being a good parent is so broad, so all encompassing, that it's impossible to measure. Being a good parent is subjective. It requires opinion, not fact, and subjectivity is somewhat rubbery: we can stretch it quite a bit in any direction.

Worry Circle issues that people can influence but cannot control are categorized as uncontrollable because the stresses cannot be remedied by personal action. So, there's no point in carrying the emotional burden. Let the others own their own solutions.

Influence issues should never be worried about in their entirety, since doing so brings a heavy, uncontrollable emotional burden. These must be dissected, to define the boundaries of what portion of a worry can be controlled by our actions.

Jettison the rest. Never carry the total weight of an issue you can only influence. Doing so is pointless.

Referring back to the parenting example, what elements of effective parenting can we control? Perhaps things like: Are we a good role model? Are we accessible every day, devoting undivided attention to our child? Do we listen? Do we teach? Do we lead by example? Do we demonstrate good habits around the child, and never bad ones? Each of these questions is answerable with a fact-based "yes" or "no," meaning it is objective and measurable rather than subjective and opinionated. In this example, we own our behaviors and we don't stress about the millions of choices our child hypothetically might make.

Things We Can't Influence or Control

According to my research, nearly two out of every five Worry Circle issues are unsolvable wastes of time and energy!

This is dangerous for huge reasons, because of the vulnerable way our mind treats worry. When we worry about things beyond our control, we tend to dwell on them to the worst possible extreme (which is most unlikely to ever happen). Our mind races in helter-skelter, panic, despair, and futility. For example, what if a corporate cutback causes a mandatory reduction in force and you suddenly lose your job? Your mind might rocket through the worst possible scenarios:

- The job market's horrible. Nobody's hiring. You'll never get another job.
- You won't be able to dump your house. The market's too

bad. Banks aren't lending and nobody's buying. You're trapped, doomed. Without a job, you'll fall behind in the mortgage payments, lose the house, and all your possessions. You'll be homeless.

- Having lost the house, you'll lose your health insurance. Then you'll get sick and need a serious operation. Your savings will be wiped out. You'll plunge into hock beyond your ability to ever recover. You'll be bankrupt, tin-panhandling busted.

- Your spouse won't stick around, will leave you, and take the kids. Who could blame them? Who'd want a loser like you?

- You'll be sued for child support. Without a job, you won't be able to pay. You'll never be able to pay. A deadbeat panhandler, out on the street. WILL WORK FOR FOOD. All Santa will bring is a cardboard square and a black magic marker.

- Because you can't pay support, you'll get arrested. Then go to jail. Heaven knows what would happen there. Even worse, your kids will resent and disown you.

This cerebral phenomenon—worrying about uncontrollable things in their worst possible extreme—is behaviorally predictable and forges a vital life lesson: When we focus on things we *can't* control, we dwell on them ceaselessly and open ourselves to severe emotional vulnerability. We trade logic and confidence for uncertainty and panic. This is a very bad neighborhood for our mind to visit.

Spiraling overreactions flood the brain with negative energy that provides no solution. The mind races in wild tangents, to ultimate boundless extremes. The big question, of course, is *why*? The short answer is we haven't learned a better way—yet!

Aside from wasted time, stress, and stewing over uncontrollable issues, these worries take a cumulative toll on the mind and body. Chronic worriers get beaten down: emotionally wounded, physically weakened, and eventually exhausted. They are susceptible to far more serious problems and depression.

Crushed under the weight of "what if" creates collateral damage, too, affecting those with whom we live, work, and care about. Some people snap, lashing out at family or society.

There is a way out. To avoid the problems that come from embracing every conceivable worry, we learn to manage our thoughts, with discipline. If our behavior can create a solution, we can take ownership of the problem. If our behavior can't change it, we don't allow the thought to stay between our ears.

It's important to be the custodian of our thoughts. To filter what comes in, accept worries we can do something about. Sweep out what doesn't.

Our mind isn't a waiting room for chaos. To be happy and balanced, we police our thoughts—with discipline.

People who are happy and centered have a strong command of their Worry Circle. They only think about what they have the power to remedy. They operate from a position of confidence.

When our mind and heart are a boiling cauldron of things

we can't control, our happiness and confidence fluctuate. When problems are bigger than us and bigger than our ability to solve them, it's easy to feel overrun. Never get there. Never get trapped into feeling helpless or overwhelmed.

If you ever do, write down what's eating at you. Sort the issues out—into all three categories. Own what you can change. Get rid of the rest.

With command of our Worry Circle, we're better able to avoid mood swings and stay centered. If we manage our worries, we aren't vulnerable to emotional upheavals and duress. Be one of those. Accept as worries only the 62 percent within your control. The other two out of five worries have no place in your mind at all!

Worrying about uncontrollable things wastes time, saps positive energy, and converts a series of thoughts into a puddle of emotional stress. With discipline, we know what worries to reject. This gives us a stronger emotional balance. The key is *choosing* what we think about … *refusing* to allow in what we can do nothing about.

Noise is only noise if we hear it. Effective Worry Circle management is policing our thoughts—keeping the noise out. The result is stronger emotional positioning. Do this every day and it becomes a habit. As it does, we grow stronger.

Stress (and depression) can begin over something small. Unbridled stress stores worries, swells, triples in size, and eventually can put us flat on our back because our health and well-being take a hit; so do our self-image and self-esteem.

When the pluses in our mind are greater than the minuses, overall we feel good. When the negatives outweigh the positives, we feel down.

Worry Circle management enables us to maximize the positives and minimize the negatives. It's a *process* to secure our thoughts, so the right thoughts stay in, and the wrong ones we eradicate.

To recap:

- We continually face three types of worries: things we can control, things we can only influence, and things we cannot control.
- We own the worries we can control, but block the rest.
- When we handle our worries appropriately, we minimize our emotional burdens.

None of us will ever stop worrying, but we can protect our life balance and happiness by *choosing* what we will and will not worry about. The downside of getting overrun by worry is enormous. Left to fester, worry quickly transforms into a monster. All we have to learn is: We can *change* what we worry about. We can police what's permitted to loiter between our ears and reject other possible worries. We can learn to let worries go. The following chapters offer tools for exactly how to do this.

What has life put between yours ears? To find out what's bugging you, refer back to the exercise at the start of this chapter. The objective of Exercise #2 is to sort the contents of the large circle in Exercise #1 into the two circles marked C ("controllable") and U ("uncontrollable").

Issues that you can remedy by your own actions are controllable. If you can only influence an issue, or not control it at all, route it into the "uncontrollable" circle.

Chances are you have worries in both categories, C and U. Sorting them enables you to instantly see what you can change for the better, and what to eradicate from your thoughts.

You may feel you have a universe of worries in your mind. When an issue becomes important enough to deal with, deal with it. This action alone will give you control. Don't worry about something until you need to make the choice—deal with it or let it go. Kick out all the uncontrollables.

Whatever remains in your controllable circle, *own it!* Want it to go away? You are empowered to erase it. Take whatever actions you need in order to resolve the problem.

Next, we'll look at where worries come from, the six most common categories.

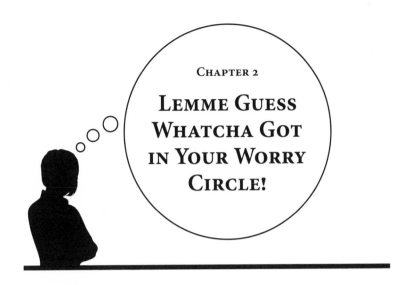

Chapter 2

Lemme Guess Whatcha Got in Your Worry Circle!

Worry isn't always bad. Sometimes it's a good thing, because it can spur us to take action. When inspired, we attack new challenges and achieve new heights. But if we don't have discipline about what we will or will not worry about, we can carry the weight of the world.

Excessive worry is counter-productive. We must have a filtration process to deal smartly with the myriad of distractions that pop into our head. Unchecked, the emotional static from rampant worry crackles loudly. Conversely, when we police our thoughts (manage our Worry Circle) we are able to focus solely on concerns that do deserve our time and emotional energy. Sorting this out is a learned behavior. Part of the process is becoming aware of the six common categories we worry about.

What DO People Worry About?

What categories frequently cause us to worry? People worry about three *types* of things: what they can control, what they can influence, and what they cannot control. These worries usually fall into six broad categories, each with its own subset issues, which are detailed in the chapters that follow. The six categories are:

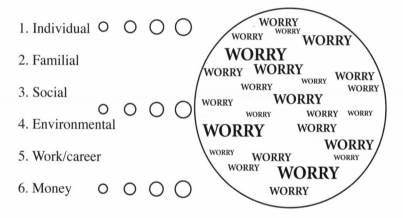

1. Individual

2. Familial

3. Social

4. Environmental

5. Work/career

6. Money

The Common Thread: Change to the Status Quo

When powerless to combat forced change, don't waste time trying. Embrace it. For example, while technological gimmickry and the information avalanche have caused behavioral chaos, like it or not, fans of old ways of communicating must adapt. Handwritten letters are dinosaurs. So are newspapers. May they rest in peace, some day to be discovered and studied by social archeologists.

Change usually creates more good than bad, but how we feel about it relies somewhat on how we choose to see it. When we view change as good, it's easy to embrace. When we see it as the enemy, we'll struggle. The reason for this is simple. The mind travels through four distinct emotional steps when processing a significant change:

(1) First, the need to change, which typically evolves over time.

(2) Panic arrives—the moment a change becomes reality. We want peace of mind, which comes only from fully understanding how a change will affect us personally. Rather than be rational about this, many people fear that everything is theoretically possible and, suspecting the worst, spiral out in uncontrollable worry. Daggers are poised to strike from every shadow. During the panic stage, we are too emotional to process our thoughts logically. Until that emotion is defused (in stage three, Acceptance), we struggle to embrace the new reality.

(3) The acceptance stage is trading emotion for logic. We have accepted a change and how it may impact us. Now we refocus away from our wild stress, toward operating within new rules and boundaries.

(4) The flourish stage enables us to match our talents with our challenges, so we may thrive. Flourishing is a great place to be, so it's smart to embrace change quickly.

The Four Stages of Change

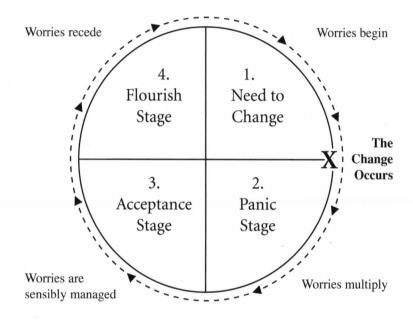

Managing Change: *The better you do it, the fewer Worry Circle issues your mind will generate.*

It's normal to have a selfish motivation when a change mandate comes down. It's smart to know the four stages of change, to move quickly from panic to acceptance, and to strive to flourish under the new conditions.

If we dwell in the panic stage, our Worry Circle overflows. For the most part, our Worry Circle is filled with things we can't control, which makes worrying a counterproductive waste of time and an emotional drain. Realizing that the four-step emotional passage is normal helps us to smartly manage change. Making the jump from panic to acceptance is vital. The sooner we do it, the faster we can regain positive traction.

Moving quickly through panic and acceptance, we leave behind the worst cause of worry: overreaction. Acceptance creates clarity, raw emotions are replaced by logic, and worry issues diminish. We shift from being out of balance to back in balance. A very good place to be.

The bigger a change, the more important is communication. Barack Obama's presidential campaign fully applied this fundamental management principle. His team sold a promise of safe change by blanketing the nation with echoing electronic messages (digital and video). This strategy netted seventy million voters and three-quarters of a billion dollars in campaign donations. Most importantly, Obama's relentless electronic urging to embrace change netted him the presidency. His team sold the concept that change was needed ... and safe. His speeches dwelled on stage three "acceptance" and what change could mean for America. This terrific politicking netted Barack

Obama the White House.

The four-stage emotional transformation requires embracing change in the right way: to manage the Worry Circle effectively (especially during Panic), to remain poised and balanced as ramifications of change unfold.

Strength comes from within. By minimizing what, and how long, we'll worry about the variables of change, our power grows from being centered and in balance—even when others around us are screaming during the world's newest amusement ride: the financial rollercoaster.

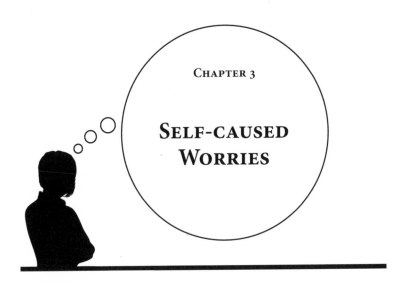

CHAPTER 3

SELF-CAUSED WORRIES

Mortality is very inconvenient. It often ruins otherwise perfect weekends. From time to time, all of us are forced to deal with things like:

- *Physical problems.* The medical industry is like Las Vegas. It exists for a reason, and we're the ones who fund it.

- *Hormonal chemistry.* Puberty, PMS, post-partum depression, and menopause all create stress that manifests into Worry Circle issues. Handle them respectfully and own the behaviors that stem from dealing with them.

- *Emotional rollercoasters.* Success and failure force decisions, often big ones (or a series in quick succession). Forced decisions commonly cause worry.

- *Cognitive limitations.* Poor concentration and reduced attention span cause stressful situations, as does the indecision they create ("paralysis by analysis"). This includes a steadily rising number of chronic digital behavioral addictions (text and email dependency), their impact on changing habits, and the worries they spawn from misinterpreted messages.
- *Frustrations.* Superman is a fictional character. Don't use him as your role model, nor put too much pressure on yourself. All you'll do is weaken two sources of strength: your self-image and self-esteem. Both are vulnerable to kryptonite.

Following are two quick exercises. Take a few minutes to complete them.

Exercise #1. Write five things that accurately describe what you believe are true about you.

1.

2.

3.

4.

5.

Exercise #2. Write five things that accurately describe how you feel about yourself.

1.

2.

3.

4.

5.

These two simple exercises shed light on potential *self-caused* Worry Circle issues by inspecting your self-esteem and self-image. In Exercise #1 you described your self-image, what you think about yourself. In Exercise #2, you shed light on your self-esteem, how you feel about yourself.

Since Worry Circle issues are emotional *conclusions*, their existence results from a compilation of thoughts. Often, our personal worries stem from conflicts or compromises. To minimize Worry Circle issues caused by self-esteem shortcomings, it's important to understand where worries come from.

Typically worries stem from three inner conflicts: how we *want* to be perceived by others, how we *are* perceived, and who we really are.

To minimize our self-esteem worries, we do ourselves a big favor when we become ultra-comfortable in our own skin: We are enthused about what we believe is true about us. We feel good about who we are. We exude positive energy. People see self-confidence in us and respond supportively.

Impatience is another source of worry. If you find that impatience is a catalyst for your own irritation and impatience, take note. Contentment doesn't blossom from instant gratification, which seemed to be a drug of choice during the economy's long run-up.

Each of us has a varying degree of mental strength. Some folks are tougher between the ears than others. Our upbringing and significant emotional events have a lot to do with whether we are resilient. Someone who's lived a lifetime of entitlement isn't as tough as someone knocked down a dozen times en route to becoming a self-made success.

Significant Emotional Events

Our upbringing shapes our core beliefs. Significant emotional events change our values and how we look at the world as we age. Episodes of life, both good and bad, arrive in sudden and unpredictable ways and rock our status quo. These events can be wonderful or devastating and traumatic. They can be controllable or uncontrollable. They do happen—to us and to others. Examples include winning a lottery, getting married, landing a new job with a big raise or mandatory relocation, a sudden illness, a physical or emotional attack, a serious accident, the birth or loss of a child.

Significant emotional events can be thrust upon us, or we can create them in the lives of others—and they land with a resounding impact. How we deal with them shapes and reshapes who we are. They are a huge source of Worry Circle angst.

Because of their hard-hitting intensity, such worries must be corralled quickly and monitored continuously. It's important to work swiftly to control our emotions (otherwise they control us).

Life-changing events are inevitable, so it's vital to recognize how they can impact our Worry Circle and how best to deal with them. If not, the merry-go-round of worry can imprison us.

Self-generated Pressures

Many life pressures are symptomatic of oversubscribed and super-busy people. Tense and hurried "Get it done, not right" is most common with Type A personalities, who are active, animated, and outgoing. Some workaholics seem to thrive on chaos.

Nevertheless, overdoing leads to anxiety, which leads to negative thinking, and worriers are susceptible to dwelling on hypothetical and uncontrollable concerns. Type B personalities are more internalized and less frantic.

Regardless of our personal style, we must own our behavioral choices and not fret over the small stuff. If the small stuff grows into something sizeable that matters, however, don't mess around. Deal with it, bury it, and move on.

Bad habits, old and new, cause worry, often from guilt. Aside from undesirable, ill-advised "sin" behaviors, depending upon our personality, we might watch the impact of less obvious choices like caffeine, salt, and sugar. Caffeine amps us up and increases our susceptibility to being irritable. Salt often increases blood pressure. Sugar gives us a "jump," soon followed by a "crash." Moderation helps, as does staying fit. Obesity pressures worry the body, tarnishing our self-image and self-esteem.

Here's a sample list of challenging Worry Circle stress triggers. Some are biggies. *All* can be tightly managed.

- Bad, dumb, or embarrassing behavior (perhaps causing humiliation or arrest). Once may be an accident, twice a coincidence, but three is a trend. Watch out.
- Legal entanglements. Lawyers work like white-collar taxis. Billable hours add up fast and freak people out.
- Minor law violations (e.g., traffic ticket). Flashing lights in the rearview mirror? *Nuts!*
- Poor decision-making. To paraphrase the immortal boxer Joe Louis: We can run from our conscience, but we

cannot hide.

- Unexpected pregnancy (to you or by you).
- Worsening of your health; doubly-so if self-induced.
- Significant increase or loss of personal wealth. (Never keep score this way, or your Worry Circle issues will bubble over.)
- Sexual frustrations or difficulties.
- Changing habits (e.g., smoking, exercise, eating, loss of sleep, erratic mealtimes, cessation of hobbies).
- Feeling unattractive (e.g., undesired weight gain).
- Drug and/or alcohol problems.
- Failure to meet personal goals.
- Failure to meet obligations.
- Vacation, especially with extended family.
- Travel, especially when on the road too often for too long (a nomadic existence).

These stress triggers range in size from inconvenient to forever life-changing. The common thread is that all are completely or at least partially controllable. We can own all or a portion of how we handle whatever each issue creates. Or we can slough off and disregard elements over which we have no control.

Personal issues like these require our *ongoing* emotional grooming. Grab the worry. Filter it as controllable, influenceable, or uncontrollable. Take action accordingly.

Stress triggers do not go away on their own. The quickest

way to retire them from the Worry Circle is to step up, own what we should, and take action—now. (Procrastination is the enemy. It gives worries time to grow out of control.)

Oversubscription

In our technology-fueled era, we are relentlessly busy. Super people! Overcommitted! A sure way to cram a Worry Circle.

Frantic and frenzied is a difficult pace to sustain. Juggling too many priorities puts pressure on us to complete too many things and please too many people. Oversubscribers self-impose a pressure to perform and are susceptible to lack of sleep, erratic eating habits, and "do-overs." When a job is done in a rush, the focus is on completing, not quality. In some businesses, that's okay. In others, it's not. Shoddy work produced in haste is totally avoidable.

For people who've grown up in what's been labeled "the entitlement generation," "helicopter parents" have hovered nearby to swoop in and protect their children. In the business world, this doesn't exist. Whoever's being paid is accountable for producing value.

A comprehensive survey a few years ago by the Sales Executive Council of the Washington, D.C.-based Corporate Executive Board showed that the number one reason good salespeople choose to leave a job is because they've stopped growing.

It's safe to assume this is why non-sales workers leave, too. Jobs get boring quickly when one's talent is underutilized or unchallenged, even in a sinking economy. People want to be valued.

If you find yourself in this type of situation, don't fuss and fume. Look at whatever elements of the situation you can control. Identify new personal-growth opportunities you *can* pursue and aggressively chase them. Don't wait!

The recent climate of dramatic corporate cutbacks choked dollars that were formerly earmarked for developing employees. Rather than stew over this global economic reality, decide what's smart to *learn*, then proactively pursue it. Don't wait for others to hand opportunities to you. Seek opportunities. Make them happen.

Invest in yourself, to more quickly separate from your competition. Accelerate toward the life you *want* to live.

The frustration of stymied personal or professional growth is very much controllable. The more aggressively we own and pursue positive personal change, the more powerful we become.

Self-caused Worry Circle issues are nearly always controllable. Don't fear them. Step up and deal with them … and keep on moving.

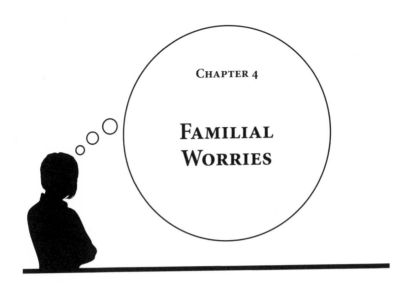

CHAPTER 4

FAMILIAL WORRIES

Relationship conflict with a spouse, partner, kids, or in-laws is as much a part of life as sunrises and sunsets. Family dynamics are a common source of worry. Nuclear families are exceedingly tough, especially during the assimilation stage. Drawing a parallel to business management, nuclear families are "born, form, storm, and then perform." Born from love. Formed by assemblage. Stormed through ground rules, boundaries, space, and other arguments. Finally, after all that, they perform as a team.

Sometimes we can influence a family issue—but not control it. We can control *our* portion. We must block out the rest.

This is difficult for parents who cling to second-guessing and emotional ownership when their kids fall victim to drugs, alcohol, bad influences, or illness. We can't own someone else's problem, and it does no good to pretend we can. Own your own behaviors ... and no more. Being a martyr benefits no one.

Common familial Worry Circle triggers include parental, spousal, sibling, and child issues; such as related to mortality, marriage, maternity, changing dynamics, social interactions, and finances.

Mortality Issues

These often tie to the worsening of a family member's health or the loss of a loved one, whether expected or unexpected. During this emotional and traumatic time, managing our Worry Circle can help us stay strong while others around us are panicking. What *can* you control when dealing with a family member's illness? Your behaviors. Your support. What *can't* you control? Their affliction.

Knowing the difference between empathy and sympathy helps. Empathy enables us to identify with and relate to another person's feelings and troubles. Sympathy is an expression of pity or sorrow for the other person's duress. Empathy helps. Sympathy doesn't. Empathy is supportive. Sympathy triggers Worry Circle issues in the mind of the afflicted.

Death is tough to deal with, because the book is closed on the relationship. There is no going back, no fixing, no clarifying, no apologizing.

We assume a natural order to life: old people passing away, babies taking their place. A young person dying disrupts our sense of right and balance with a resounding emotional shock that challenges life's implied doctrine of fairness. The young person has been cheated out of the right to grow old.

How can we manage the Worry Circle of death? Remember the four stages of change. Stage two (Panic) is the emotional trauma we feel when someone has died. It's normal to be upset. We don't let go and move on until we reach stage three (Acceptance). When we honor the deceased and remember all that's good, we reach the acceptance stage. When we let it, time can soften the pain.

Marital Issues

This category includes spousal friction, separation, divorce (especially acrimonious), and remarriage. In tough economic times, strong families draw closer. Others convert their stress into increased marital friction.

Friction (fighting). This is the behavioral reaction to an emotional manifestation of negative thought. The thought(s) may be accumulated or spontaneous. From a Worry Circle perspective, what's the best way to react? Work backwards. Logic cannot overlay emotions, so both combatants need to diffuse their emotions in order to logically discover and discuss their reasoning.

What we think drives how we feel. How we feel drives what we do. So, progress comes from understanding each other's collected thoughts.

When arguing, strive to retire emotion from the conflict as soon as possible. Focus on the thoughts that shaped the emotion that caused the person's reaction. Since it's pointless to argue over emotions, seek the *reasons* the other person feels the way he or she does. One properly phrased question could do the trick: "Well, it's obvious this is upsetting you. What thoughts are causing you to feel this way?"

Separation. The same approach holds true when dealing with marital separation. Remember, separation is a choice, acted on due to an emotional conclusion by one or both parties: (1) Personal comfort will improve. Life will get better by being apart. (2) Separating will keep things from getting worse, reduce the heavy toll and emotional burden. We prefer to do what it will take to avoid the situation getting progressively worse.

To manage our Worry Circle, we seek to understand *why* this has come about. Until the thoughts that fueled the impetus to leave are discussed, there is little chance the relationship will recover.

During additional heightened emotional traumas, such as the world is currently facing, it becomes more important than ever to sort out the sources of motivation and fear. For much of the past generation, we became a throwaway society. Whether a product or a relationship, when it broke we threw it away and got a new one. We stopped repairing things. A relationship isn't an old toaster. Fix it.

Divorce. Divorce is an emotional hand grenade, and the dominoes of duress seem endless. You name it—family, money, living arrangement, social assimilation—divorce disrupts it and the emotional scars cut deep.

From a Worry Circle point of view, what can be controlled during a divorce? Our own thoughts, feelings, and behaviors. Divorce is a classic, textbook example of the four-stage wheel of change in action. (1) The need to split evolves over time (stage one). (2) The hammer falls and suddenly the Worry Circle is flooded by a broken-levee of "what ifs?" which create panic (stage two), and we dwell on the gut-wrenching upheaval. For some, mourning or bitterness extends the stage of worry. (3) Until healing is done, there is no crossing over to acceptance (stage three). (4) Only when the new status quo is embraced does or can life improve (stage four, *Flourish*). Here the baggage is stored and a new, better life is underway.

The four stages of change are a process. We can go fast or slow. But one way or the other, during and following a divorce everyone makes this trek. Make a game out of it, a race to reach the acceptance stage, and life becomes a whole lot easier.

Remarriage. How do we assimilate new lovers into our life filled with other relationships? How do we get our kids to accept them? We hope for the best—acceptance of a new spouse by family members, but few are superglue-tight from the get-go.

To manage the Worry Circle, remember what causes behaviors: What we think drives how we feel, and how we feel drives what we do. When we want someone new in our life to be accepted, others must come to perceive that as good. If their thoughts are positive, acceptance will happen. If not, acceptance won't happen until those thoughts are reengineered into a more positive light.

Telling people how they're supposed to feel doesn't work.

It's like a thin sheet of ice over a cold pond of deep water.
No one likes being told what to think or how to feel. Most
resentfully push back, and do the opposite. So, we must invest
energy in building a strong platform of positive thoughts.

Remember, the introduction of a new spouse into the family
dynamic is a significant change, so the four stages of change
come into play and each family member has to make that
journey. Some circle the change wheel quickly, others slowly.
We must avoid the temptation to push everyone around at our
preferred clockspeed. Otherwise we'll meet resistance, and
arguing only escalates emotions. So, focus on managing your
own thoughts in a positive way and supporting others as they
deal with their own wheel of change.

Maternal Issues

Three dramatically different scenarios cause intense
fluctuations in baby-related, emotional amplitude:

- Pregnancy, planned for or unexpected.
- Accidental loss or personal choice to terminate a
  pregnancy.
- Troubled birth, medical complications.

The easiest thing to do is raise someone else's kid. The
hardest thing is to raise our own. However, to me, the only thing
in life that adds dimension is parenthood.

Some couples pursue this ambition with steadfast
determination. Others get the news by accident. I myself am the
byproduct of the revelry of a boisterous New Year's Eve party.
A second child, my arrival was unexpected. My parents were

forced to move from an apartment into a house, an expensive and unplanned decision.

Depending on a couple's relationship and life circumstance, stork flyovers range from euphorically good news to numbing shock. Pregnancies are forced change; managing the worries that go with them requires separating logic from emotion. Men and women sometimes travel different paths dealing with the news.

Losing a baby is, of course, radically different. Rather than building toward an impending inevitability of gain, one is forced to deal with the burden of loss. Once a pregnancy is gone, it cannot be reversed. Dwelling on "what ifs" can be debilitating.

There is comfort in relying on the four-stage wheel of change. The emotional devastation of stage two (Panic) takes time to get over. That's okay. Just stay in the present and don't get tangled in the emotional web. When the time is right, stage three (Acceptance) is waiting.

Losing a child is rated as life's greatest trauma. The loss forces one to face the heaviest emotional challenges ever. For some, the grief looms too high. Others cope by honoring their loss through devotion to help others.

Rock legend Eric Clapton made the courageous call to beat the demons of addiction to honor his lost son, Conor, who died in a fall in New York City at the age of four in 1991. Clapton had been a reluctant father and only came to realize what his son meant to him the day before his child died. For every day since then, Clapton the father has honored the memory of his son by helping thousands stay sober and overcome addiction.

Changing Dynamics

Moving away from home, by choice or necessity, is life changing, especially for the 50 percent to 70 percent of Americans who leave the town where they were born.

Moving out forces change. The parent-child relationship is altered as the offspring's self-image, self-esteem, and self-worth expand. Many children get homesick. Parents go through separation anxiety, a mid-life role reversal in direct contrast to the early years of life, when a young child panics when separated from mom.

To manage the Worry Circle, what can and cannot be changed? If the move was necessary, there's no point worrying about the good old days. Instead, focus on creating new good days.

When a major move is domestic, home may be one airplane ride away. There is comfort in knowing that if anything arises that's too big to handle alone, one quick trip to the airport can help engage the cavalry.

Long-distance international uprooting creates Worry Circle issues for the people left behind, more than for the one on the adventure. The ones behind dwell on what they've lost. The one on the road is excited about what lies ahead. Managing our worry means owning what can be controlled and dropping the rest. Sometimes we just have to let go.

In the words of former New York Yankee outfielder Mickey Rivers, a famed non-worrier of his generation, "Ain't no sense worryin' 'bout stuff you got no control over, 'cause if you got no control over it, ain't no sense worryin'."

Mickey was a fun player to watch. His common-sense philosophy perfectly describes how to deal with a long-distance separation.

Another thing that changes a family's dynamics is the sudden addition (by marriage) or subtraction (by divorce) of family members. Like-personality styles typically mesh; whereas, unlike styles typically clash. What can be managed? What we look for. When we look for what's good in another, that's what we see. When we look for what's different, *that's* what we'll see. What we choose to look for is a personal choice ... and 100 percent controllable.

Social Interactions

Put any mix of folks together because they must be there and watch the magic. Some people get along great; others go after each other like cobras and mongooses. Alcohol can be an accelerant, clashing egos. People who are comfortable with themselves have fewer issues during social interactions than those who are consumed by how they appear. Dueling martinis between caustic straight shooters causes loud disagreements. Narcissists, people in love with themselves, can't handle criticism.

Holidays, reunions, and vacations bear the brunt of egotistical swordfights. Seeing it as a game helps us understand the dynamic through the lens of others. Less judging and more tolerance minimizes the number of skirmishes. We appreciate that personal differences are fine, not threatening.

Family arguments and harboring long-term grudges do happen, because family people insist on being right (rather than accepting differences). When it comes to core beliefs and opinions, there is no right or wrong. There's only personal choice.

Fraternal conflict puzzles me, because communication problems can be fixed. My brother and I are close; but I have two friends, one in Florida, one in Kentucky, who don't speak to their brothers. All four of them are waiting for the sibling to make amends rather than talk things out. It is quite all right to have a different point of view. What is the Worry Circle remedy? Quit thinking that all issues have a right or wrong and agree to disagree. Shake hands (or hug) and let it go. Personal behavior is controllable.

Financial

Money is a Worry Circle topic unto itself (chapter eight). It can implode a family's dynamic. Change catalysts include significant increase, decrease or loss of family income, significant loss of investment value, a threatened or wiped out retirement plan.

Financial issues are a bit like fishing. When times are good, fish are everywhere. They're easy enough to catch, maybe more than we need. When bank accounts grow and portfolios expand, the fish are biting. Family members have plenty to help each other. So, when family members argue over finances, a lot of times the skirmish isn't really about the money. It's about ego. Ego is big inside the Worry Circle: *Am I good enough?*

When the economy tanked, the fish quit biting. Overnight, they disappeared. The big ones vanished. The days of plenty were gone. We could fish all day, hoping to catch something to eat, but the fish weren't where they used to be. The worry became how to find them. High tide, low tide, didn't matter. Everybody was looking but nobody was finding. Stress went up.

It sounds trite to say "It is what it is," but it's true. The rules of the economy have changed—so we need to re-broker agreements. Wailing and gnashing teeth doesn't help. It just keeps us from seeing possibilities.

The days of instant gratification are over, and worrying about the way things used to be doesn't change a thing. Rather than dwell on a fish that got away, keep fishing. Things don't change unless *we* change them.

Financially induced familial stress creates big worries, but remember: Families create heritage. Value them, protect them, strengthen them, and cherish them. Never implode the family dynamic over a business deal.

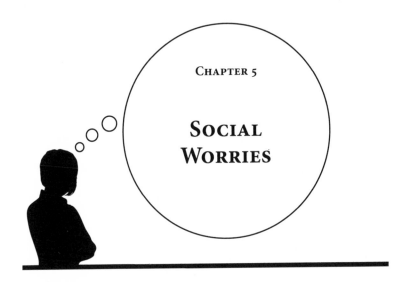

CHAPTER 5

SOCIAL WORRIES

Each of us has different interpretations of what's right or wrong with society. When we watch or read the news, it seems a lot is wrong. There *are* a lot of people hurting out there. With the economy the way it is, more are bound to follow.

Many internalize their suffering. Others vent their anguish. Road rage and air rage are dramatic social confrontations that represent emotions running amok. Some people just snap. How can *we* avoid that?

One of my closest friends, Tim Chew of Jacksonville Beach, Florida, I have bestowed with the title, World Policeman. He hates slobs, rudeness, drivers who hog two parking spaces, anyone who cuts in line, and cigarette butts flipped out car windows. When Tim is out patrolling the world, he lets offenders know.

Interacting with others does, from time to time, cause friction. This is true whether we're friends or strangers. Following are some common causes of social conflict.

Unpolished, Uncertain, or Inadequate Social Skills

The higher we aspire, the more we need social skills flexibility. In England, a gentleman uses a butter knife even when dining alone. In India, hundreds of millions of people eat righthanded, never with the left, shoveling food in with their fingers. One set of social skills doesn't fit every scenario.

Interfacing with Opposite Personality Types and Styles

People range from shy and unassertive types to bold and brash "in your face." Type A personalities are hyper. Type Bs are reserved. Type Cs are calm on the outside, agitated on the inside, and often don't openly express their feelings. Just because someone is different doesn't mean those differences are worth worrying about.

Conflicting Ambition

For many, living a life absent of fulfillment (personal, professional, or both) is a hollow existence riddled with remorse and self-doubt. For them, life might be better with a little more passion. For others, a cautious life, guarded and protected, is the safest way to live. Opposites don't always attract. Sometimes differences cause conflict.

Relationship Issues

Relationships take time—but they fill Worry Circles quickly. Family and friends all vie for attention.

One way to minimize friction caused by a misunderstanding or a difference of opinion is to resist the urge to dig in and defend a position; to waste less time judging people's behaviors as good or bad, their opinions as right or wrong. Instead, withhold judgment; and channel your energy toward listening and observing, to better understand the reasons behind their different points of view.

Our own viewpoint is not unimpeachably correct, and someone else's opposite view is not necessarily wrong. When we assume the opposite position, that another may be right and we may be wrong, we are seeing through their lens and can better understand their point of view. Even if we don't agree, at least we can understand. The better we understand, the less likely their differences will bother us.

People enter relationships with different upbringings, core beliefs, ambitions and agendas, learning and communication styles. We also have conflicting expectations, different measurement standards, and different tolerance levels (including those for risk).

In matters of the heart, someone need not always be right and the other person wrong. Life is easier when we don't always have to be right.

To strengthen a relationship, avoid the urge to dig in. Focus on the fix. Stubborn gets us nowhere. Winning isn't being right or wrong. Winning occurs when the problem goes away.

Relationships are *guaranteed* to have worries, because we are all emotionally dependent. Worry Circle issues can be all-consuming, and friction is always difficult. A broken heart is a heavy thing to carry around, especially when breaking up wasn't our idea. So, occasionally we may need to superglue our broken heart. Saying it is easier than doing it, but repairing it is better than living with it.

We tend to judge ourselves by our intentions; others judge us by our actions and achievements. Bosses don't care about our promises; nor do disappointed friends and lovers. We all go through life with a personal agenda, and no two are the same. Relationships don't always turn out the way we want, and people seldom do what we hope they will. People will do what they will do. Worrying won't change it, and it won't change them. If anything, it may push them further away.

A slew of social stimuli cause us to worry, such as:

- *Starting a serious, committed relationship.* Forsaking all others is a big choice. Some can do it. Some can't.

- *Moving in.* Within thirty days of my own marriage, my wife had replaced 96 percent of my stuff with hers. My stuff went curbside. I love my wife, but I missed my stuff.

- *Domestic arguments.* Best case, these are emotionally taxing. Worst case, emotionally debilitating, especially the ones that perpetuate.

- *Being betrayed, including physical and/or emotional infidelity.* Emotional scars take longer to heal than physical ones. They re-open easier, too.

- *Getting dumped*. Regardless of whether we are the dump-er or the dump-*ee*, it's never easy to close a life chapter and move on.
- *Breaking-up a long-term relationship*. Starting over is doubly difficult after a significant portion of life has been with someone in whom we've invested a tremendous amount of time, money, emotion, and energy. Facing the fact that he or she has no sustaining value for us is a bitter pill to swallow, but it must be done.
- *Getting married*. Some days are island sunshine, others Siberian winters. If it weren't so hard, more people would do it.
- *Marital difficulties*. They come free with the wedding dress and tuxedo. Expect troubles and deal with them—always with a goal to resolve, rather than escalate. But if your father-in-law gives you a good sofa ... take it.
- *Separation*. Doubly difficult. New physical, emotional, and financial burdens. A recent growing trend is the number of couples who want to split up but can't afford to. So, the new, tolerated relationship is: economic hostages.
- *Divorce*. If this is inevitable, keep your chin up and keep moving forward.
- *Legal and financial ramifications of the split*. It's acidic to everyone when lawyers take a third or a half of the assets the two of you worked so hard to accumulate.
- *Death of a close friend by illness, accident, or tragedy*.

A true Worry Circle test. Can't control it, can't change it. What we can control is how we choose to deal with it. One way is to remain grateful that person enriched our life.

- *Bad things happening to good people (injustices).* If you are the good person, stay positive. If it's someone else, teach him or her how to manage worries. Coach them to remain relentlessly positive.

- *Decrease in social involvement.* Being a valued part of a group helps our self-esteem. Subtract that and our self-esteem is at risk. Take action to stay engaged.

- *Arguments with roommates, close friends, or admired constituents.* Arced wires spark. I'm a horseman and one of my close friends, Lonnie Owens, has taught me a lot about the horse business. It's never easy to make a profit buying, breeding, or selling a racehorse. When you buy, the horse is never cheap enough. When you sell, you never sell it high enough. One of the first lessons Lonnie taught me was never to let a friendship fall out over a horse deal. Friendships transcend money. Lonnie has another rule, the Three-Day Rule. It applies to arguments, too. When something goes wrong that bugs you, it's okay to worry about it for three days. After that, it's off limits.

- *Leading an organization or being responsible for a group of people.* A group is just a collection of people, but leading a group can cause two sources of worry. One is the burden we place on ourselves. The other, the burdens others place on us. Answer: Own what you can (thoughts, feelings, and deeds). Don't obsess about the rest.

- *Social isolation.* The Unabomber was a loner. No further comment required.
- *Feeling victimized by cronyism or ethnic, racial, religious, or sexual prejudice.* This is a tough one. When faced with these, we must have the courage and determination to think beyond them. What kind of thoughts brought us here? Perpetuating (or tolerating) worry over such things is counter-productive, unless it spurs us to change our social situation. But if we dissect the collection of thoughts that got us to this point and conclude that we are being unfairly aggrieved, it's time to do what it takes to make positive change happen. When you do, toss the noise into the trashcan of forgotten memories. Harboring grudges drains our energy and well-being.
- *Conflicting interests between major priorities* (e.g., social networks, work and career, school, church). All of these take time and battle for our attention. We're busy, seeking boundaries of comfort. Friction is the likely result. When overwhelmed, prune activities back to a prioritized list. What matters most? If you can't feel good about being somewhere, what's the point of going?

Social stresses come with social interactions. That's normal. So, keep perspective, and fix relationships when they've gone sour. We can erase them via the friendship "delete key," but do that too often and we run out of friends. Heaven forbid ending up alone.

Relationships enrich our lives. Being a throwaway society doesn't mean throwing away all the people we've known, nor everyone with whom we've had a conflict. When it comes to managing social Worry Circle issues smartly, put a priority on fixing relationships, rather than discarding them. None of us wants a lonely funeral.

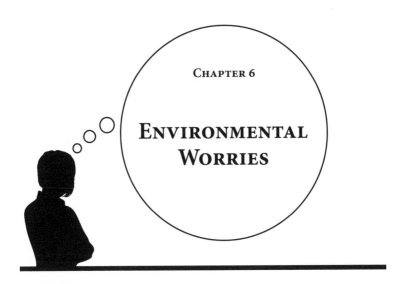

CHAPTER 6

ENVIRONMENTAL WORRIES

When I was teaching this Worry Circle program in Europe, a Serbian woman told me about her life growing up in Belgrade. Her family home had been bombed twice; fortunately, no one died. In Latvia, another student told me how her family had come to settle in Riga; her mother had escaped Siberia and, virtually indigent, had traveled secretly across Russia, desperate to gain a foothold on life. I've also spent time in Romania, where I learned of life under the communist rule of Nicolae Ceausescu.

A close friend, George Simmons, wasn't as lucky. He was killed on *9/11* by the terrorists. George and his wife were in the wrong place at the wrong time, American Airlines flight #77, skyjacked into the Pentagon. They were en route from Dulles Airport to Hawaii to spread the ashes of her late father. Instead, seven months later, a couple dozen of us poured George and

Diane's ashes into the Potomac River.

Values formed during our upbringing grind the lens through which we look at life and set into place our social norms: where we stand on issues, how important we perceive those issues, our tolerance for worry. We can control where we live, what we do for a living, and what we do in life. When life's logistics are broken (e.g., location, neighborhood, cost of living, commuting) we can study the pluses and minuses of taking action. Perhaps it's possible to eliminate a pestering negativity.

Typical environmental worries:

- *Decrease in quality of living conditions.* When it's time to go, the Worry Circle remedy is quit thinking about it. Tie your shoelaces tight and go.

- *Increase in cost of living.* A major stressor in dense, expensive cities like London, Moscow, New York City, and Tokyo. The more things cost, the more trade-offs we must make.

- *Moving and re-assimilating* (same city, out of town, out of state—all of these). If moving by choice, it's not as big a deal as if there's no option. The Worry Circle is what we make of it. Look for good, see good. Look for bad, see bad. We can control what we look for.

- *Moving to a different country.* This can be invigorating, if you speak the language; intimidating if you don't. Assimilation isn't delivered to the front door. You must immerse in order to achieve it.

- *Noisy, unfriendly, or sloppy roommate or neighbor.*

What can we control? Lead by example, coach toward positive improvement, hope for the best. If nothing changes, don't dwell on it. Don't let someone else's bad habits drive you batty.

- *Changing social demographics.* Immigration was a major political issue early in the McCain-Obama presidential campaign, but shifted to back-burner the moment the economy hit the skids. People move to certain places for certain reasons and leave for other ones. Ethnic neighborhoods are popular because people like to live among people like themselves. Don't fret changes in society.

- *Traffic and commuting.* Study the faces on commuter trains and what do you see? Zombies in neckties. The same with a choked highway, cars creeping bumper-to-bumper during killer commutes. From a time-management point of view, we all require a certain amount of time to shuttle to and from work. How we use that time—spend it, waste it, invest it, or cherish it—is a choice.

- *Less physical or personal space.* Changes to our norm are disruptive. The thought of trading our freedom for a locked jail cell six-by-seven feet by eight-feet high is strong enough to keep most of us marching the straight and narrow.

- *Substandard air quality (pollution).* I coached baseball in southern India on an open field next to a massive crematorium that belched dime-sized ash flakes out of a huge smokestack. The Indians never noticed it. For me, inhaling was tough for reasons beyond simply the physical.

- *Altitude.* Sherpas zoom up and down Mount Everest as climbing guides because they can deal with the skinny oxygen on the mountain that soars nearly six miles high. Flatlanders who play shuffleboard in Sarasota would struggle.
- *Poor water quality.* Without potable drinking water, our health and lives are in danger. This Worry Circle issue impacts how and where billions of people live. According to the United Nation, about 1.2 billion are forced to live without access to clean drinking water.
- *Climate* (rain, temperature, humidity). The saying in Seattle is if you can survive your second July there, you'll make it. It's gray and rainy half the year, glorious the other half. On the coasts, Easterners are fine with humidity, westerners abhor it. Changes to whatever we're used to require an adjustment.
- *Incurable diseases (e.g. terminal cancer, ALS).* When someone we know and care about is afflicted with a death sentence, an unchecked Worry Circle overflows.

The biggest differences I've seen between American and European workers in the years I've shuttled back and forth are the European workforce's courage and relative portability.

The long list above is a virtual checklist of reasons for exodus for billions of ambitious workers around the globe. Once the formation of the European Union opened borders for simplified European migration, millions decided to leave home with hopes of carving out a better life. They arrived as outsiders at destinations full of strangers, in different cultures with people who spoke unfamiliar languages. For most, a new life begins at the bottom, and it's a very slow climb. Their courage and fortitude is inspiring.

Many environmental worries are fixable. All it takes is courage and a willingness to embrace change.

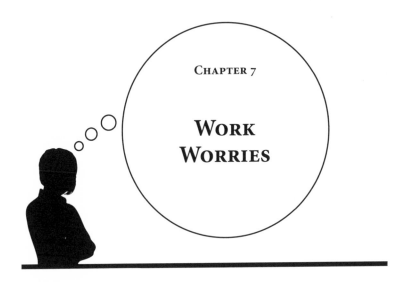

CHAPTER 7

WORK WORRIES

Work comes with built-in noise. Since a lifetime of work manufactures a whirlpool of Worry Circle concerns, it's noble to manage these distractions with minimum impact.

Work burdens create ancillary sources of angst, like changes in eating, exercising, and sleeping habits—all of which are controllable, by recalibrating our behaviors into the changing demands of our job. Modify our consumption, work to be fit, get plenty of rest. The television is not a blood relative. It doesn't care about us; nor should we care about it.

Common sources of work-related stress:

- The Job
- Co-workers
- The Boss
- The Company

The Job

Common sources of job-related worries are:

- *Ending an old job, or beginning a new one.* Closing a chapter disrupts the status quo, because starting a new one comes with a self-induced pressure to succeed.

- *Being fired or laid-off, voluntarily or involuntarily.* In a boom economy, losing a job is no big deal, because finding another is relatively easy. In a bust economy, worries are like images in the rearview mirror: they're larger than they appear.

- *Expectations to perform at a sustained high level after demonstrating success.* Sometimes this is "performance punishment," where the better we are at something, the more we have to do it. When the economy contracts, the pressure to perform expands, and pressure percolates worries.

- *Too many or too few work hours.* Work too much and we burn out. Work too little and we fret.

- *Increased or reduced responsibility.* With job enhancement comes job stress. With job contraction comes diminished value. Both create worry.

- *Feeling insecure and underqualified for what you are actually doing.* The Peter Principle: Everyone rises to the level of his or her incompetence. When *we* feel this, others can see it. If they see it, they talk about it. Nothing good grows from an incompatible reality. Only action makes this feeling disappear. Work urgently to close the gaps you sense.

- *Feeling overqualified; being bored at work and with work.* Being overqualified is often a political threat to others, which increases our own vulnerability to being replaced. Boredom is a conclusion, reached after processing too many thoughts. Don't waste your life in a dead-end situation.

- *Pressure and deadlines, real or self-imposed.* Sometimes we need to push back on being overburdened by unrealistic expectations, either our own or others of us. The moment we accept tight finishes, we worry about them. When stressful deadlines create a workload that exceeds your capacity, training, or skill set, call a time out. Unachievable deadlines take us down. Don't fear pushing back.

- *Juggling multiple priorities.* Who is more impressive: a juggler skillfully wheeling three balls in the air, or a juggler repeatedly dropping four? Protect your work quality, and don't overcommit.

- *Role ambiguity.* Overcommit or underdeliver, and we're vulnerable. Not 100 percent sure what's expected of you? Don't accept that. If you do, you'll worry about having to guess. Step up and address it. The same holds true for conflicting demands or being "dumped on." Consistently deliver what's expected in a professional way and you will be admired.

When Is It Time to Switch Jobs?

Almost overnight, the sliding economy changed the job-hopping luxury of dissatisfied workers. Today, having fewer options is unfortunate. A worker's tolerance level tends to rise along with the unemployment rate.

Since we find in life what we look for, it's important to look for the good in what we do. All around the world, people are about 93 percent the same and are inherently good. Celebrate that and ignore the rest. "No stinkin' thinkin'," as my late friend George Simmons was fond of saying.

If you can't ignore the negative noise of your current situation, try to block it out. If you can't, minimize it to the extent you can ... and remind yourself not to dwell on it.

My pal George excelled at coaching people through potential job and career changes. "Ask yourself two questions," he'd say. "Do you enjoy what you're doing? Are you fairly paid for what you do?"

If you answer yes and yes, he advised, stay put.

If you answer no and yes, can the no be turned into a yes? If there's a way, do it. If the no can't be changed, you have a choice: Is the no so vital that you can't reconcile it and put it aside? If so, it's time to seek another opportunity. If the no isn't that big a deal, ignore it (remove it from the Worry Circle) and focus only on the positives of your current position.

If you answer no and no to George's two questions—you don't like your job, and you aren't fairly paid—quit moaning and take accelerated action to change your situation. Worry Circle remedies reside in our own behaviors. What we *choose* to do in life is up to us.

It's important to note George's phraseology: "Are you *fairly* paid for what you do?" He didn't say underpaid. The problem isn't always how much we make; sometimes it's what we spend. Switching jobs may not remedy that.

It does take courage to walk away and start something new. For some, it takes more courage than they've got. If that's you, recognize and accept that, and don't browbeat yourself. Also, realize you no longer have a reason to whine about the less-than-perfect situation.

My consulting work has taken me around the world and I can assure you: A lot more people know what they *don't* want to do in life than what they truly do. Job contentment (or lack thereof) is a global malady. Most of us must work, so we face a choice: do something we love to do, or something we loathe, or something in-between. When the economy is in a state of flux, the "in-between" toleration sector gets pretty crowded.

Worries caused by transition are common. What made you great at your last job might not matter in your new responsibility. It's natural to fret about this, because we want to make a good impression.

Every job requires three things for strong, sustained performance: knowledge, skills, and attributes. Knowledge is what we know (relative to what we need to know) in order to succeed. Skills are our demonstrated ability to deliver desired results. Attributes are the intangibles that make each of us unique.

When thrust into a transition (by choice or necessity), don't panic! Also, don't let pride slow you down. Channel energy to gap-close whatever is required that is new or unfamiliar: more knowledge, new skills. If you need help, get it. You'll reduce your number of Worry Circle issues.

When we commit to doing our absolute best, and make a game of it, the game overtakes the worry. Commit to getting stronger. How quickly can you become terrific?

Co-workers

Can't everyone play in the sandbox? Co-workers, subordinates; policies and politics, HR issues (whether justified or unfair)—all blend into worry. To hear less co-worker noise, remain deaf to rumors and allergic to innuendos, because both expand the Worry Circle.

Everybody who works has some personal political agenda. In tough economic times, agendas incorporate a survival instinct. Co-workers who used to be trusted and team-oriented can morph into smiling, venomous snakes. All it takes is one hot rumor of an impending layoff.

To manage your Worry Circle, remember the cardinal rule: *All we can control is our own behaviors.* So, don't get sucked into the quicksand of rumor, gossip, and backstabbing. If someone says or does something that bugs you, confront it head on. Suppress emotion and manage by fact.

Many people worry so much about confrontation that

they'll do almost anything to avoid it. But if a conflict lingers, it festers ... and that grows the Worry Circle. When a conflict arises, spoken or unspoken, deal with it. The sooner you do, the sooner the Worry Circle issues will diminish, and possibly even evaporate.

The newest arsonist that torches co-worker relationships masquerades as a keyboard. Misunderstandings between co-workers run rampant for those who insist on typing messages that convey emotion. Avoid thumb wars. Digital exchanges at the expense of a face-to-face discussion or a phone call are silly. Mayhem spawned from emails or text messages misinterpreted by the receiver cause mix-ups because typed notes are solely word-reliant; they provide no non-verbal clues or voice inflection or tone.

In face-to-face interpersonal exchanges, 55 percent of a message is conveyed non-verbally; 38 percent is based on voice and tone; only 7 percent is the words. Because digital messages are so widely misinterpreted, the needless Worry Circle explosions they create are completely preventable. Don't let digital exchanges stew. Pick up the phone and sort things out.

The Boss

Problems with the boss are common, so never enter a job expecting otherwise. It's a heck of a lot easier to be a sole contributor than bossing around a slew of individuals under the guise of teamwork. Problems stem from:

- *Lack of recognition, formal or informal, for doing good*

work. Workers thrive on recognition. Even though it can
be free, some bosses are flat-out lousy at it.

- *Lack of respect*. We all want to feel valued. If you don't,
call a timeout and talk about it. Or else it will fester in
your Worry Circle.

- *Issues or conflicts with the boss or management*. Bosses
have businesses to run. They look at life through a
different lens than the workers. Workers value effort;
bosses value results. Bosses judge us by our behaviors,
our accomplishments, sometimes our failures. This is
why performance appraisals are stressful; stressful to
give, worse to receive.

- *A good boss isn't always a nice person*. Nice is terrific,
but results matter more. If the boss can't get results,
he or she will be replaced by someone who can. In a
tight economy, the boss has an expanded Worry Circle.
Sometimes, as the worker, it helps to step back and
worry less about the boss by re-channeling gratitude to
the fact that we have a job.

- *Lousy communication causes misunderstandings*.
Some people are better communicators than others.
If poor communication is causing you to worry, don't
swallow it. Address it. Improving communication and
understanding are very controllable.

- *Crossed wires*. Adults tend to process ideas in one of
two ways, detail-to-concept or concept-to-detail. Detail-
to-concept thinkers are methodical and systematic

in reviewing data and deriving conclusion; like an accountant, who compiles, sorts, calculates, and studies data to derive a conclusion. Whereas, concept-thinkers grab the big picture (the concept) and work backward, seeking only as much information as they need. Too much information is boring.

It's easy to see how concept thinkers would struggle with detail thinkers and vice-versa. Like styles get along fine, but opposite styles struggle. When the boss is a detail freak and you aren't, friction can develop. If you are the detail person and the boss is high-concept, he or she may get frustrated with the time you invest to painstakingly prepare support data they don't want or need.

If you have a communication problem with your boss, don't ignore it or stew over it. Try to figure out *why* the problem arose. To solve it, one of you will have to "flex" your style. A detail person presents comprehensive information, step by logical step. A conceptual thinker reacts positively to ideas, first in summary. Whatever your boss's style, try to mirror it. Package and present however much supporting information he or she requires.

If no one changes behaviors, if you insist on being detail-oriented while the boss prefers a conceptual summary (or vice-versa), you can't maximize the relationship. "Flexing" your style helps to minimize a misunderstanding, so your Worry Circle issues can disappear. No sense worrying if you don't have to.

If your boss is overly demanding, or frequently drops last-

minute emergencies in your lap, focus on the facts. Sanitize
emotion out of it. Bridge the gap between your workload and
what is realistically doable. If you don't speak up, you'll be
exposed to unfair criticism. Don't risk it. Negotiate a realistic
expectation.

In my leadership classes, we cover the three causes of
worker non-performance: either someone can't do it, won't do it,
or is prevented from doing it. A good boss delegates, empowers,
and holds the employees accountable. This requires making
sure that the workload is within the worker's capability; and
the worker should clearly understand what will be considered a
successful result.

Many folks who are promoted from worker to manager have
little experience or skills at leading people. If that's your boss,
don't expect him or her to be perfect. Job title, qualifications, and
performance don't always mesh. If you work for a good leader,
be grateful.

The Company

Jobs come, jobs go. Unless you work for yourself or a safe
branch of government, long gone are loyal careers of three-
decade allegiance, sentimental retirement parties, engraved
wristwatches. The job market is in accelerated change, due to
a sagging global economy, relentless evolving technology, an
impatient and mobile workforce, and changing demographics.

Common company-related worries are:

- *Little or no opportunity for advancement.* There's only

one way out of a dead-end job. Listen to your soul.
Change jobs. The longer you put it off, the more you'll
tarnish your self-esteem and confidence.

- *Cultural* (philosophical) *differences.* Company cultures
  vary dramatically, and cultural misfits don't belong; they
  stick out like Martians. In tight economic times, these
  people are the first culled in the downsizing.

- *Frequent rumors, re-orgs, and cutbacks.* These are
  uncontrollable, so ignore them. They are banned from
  the Worry Circle.

- *Losing a job or changing jobs* (forced or voluntary).
  Every job we ever had we were looking for at the time.
  We'll find the next one, too. Even so, people worry
  like crazy when they lose a job. It is stressful, no doubt
  about it. To manage the Worry Circle, invest every spare
  moment in the hunt—and make it an adventure. After
  all, you are searching for the buyer of the best product of
  all—you!

- *A heel-dragging reluctance to commit.* Every company
  has four categories of workers. One-fourth are totally
  committed, one-fourth are somewhat committed, another
  fourth are somewhat detached. The final fourth are
  completely detached and couldn't care less. They're just
  there to collect the check.

When we are uncommitted to our work, we are feeling
this place isn't "it." Non-commitment is a choice. With
that decision come controllable burdens that must be

carried around. These guilt pangs are smoke signals of impending change. One of two things will happen: We find a slot where we *can* commit, or we're bounced. Uncommitted employees are quick to go in a tight economy, so it's better to make the choice yourself than have someone else make it for you.

Companies have life cycles, about half as long as people, assuming the company survives its first three years of startup. Businesses are born of an entrepreneurial idea and determination to fill a need in the marketplace. They die at the hands of new and dynamic competitors. Many of the powerhouse brands of our parents' generation are today trivia questions.

Worrying about your company sustaining late in its life cycle is a noble waste of energy. While no company is around forever, what element of its survival can you support? Loyalty and effort, certainly, but your job is not *you*. It's how you pay the bills.

Every job has Worry Circle tentacles dangling beneath it. When the economy goes south, those tentacles inexorably lengthen—but they wrap around us only if we let them. With more gizmos and gadgets than ever, people work at a frenzied pace and are relentlessly busy. The number of truly *productive* people, upbeat and efficient, is dwindling. Remaining in control and happy when immersed in a stressful surrounding takes discipline of thoughts and feelings, plus a strong work ethic.

We can control what we do in life, and how committed we are to it. To minimize your Worry Circle distractions, stay positive and do the best you can at what you're paid to do.

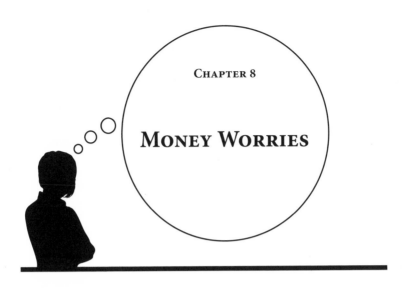

CHAPTER 8

MONEY WORRIES

"Money doesn't mean anything unless you don't have any."

— Sir Paul McCartney, billionaire musician

One person stews about money worries. Two or more argue. Money issues are wildly abundant in the Worry Circle. Have been since the day money was invented.

A bazillion things related to money bug us. The big ones are financial anxiety—the cost of living, shortfalls, and overextensions. In the world's second most expensive city, London (Moscow is first), the cost of living is the number one worry. Not surprising, since Londoners worry more than anyone else in the United Kingdom. They were good at worrying even before the banks started to teeter. Now they're terrific at it.

The economic mess of 2008 (and counting) slid us into

numerous financial concerns: income fluctuations, savings, retirement, vacations, discretionary spending. Market forces have influenced all of these. Peripheral concerns are unexpected surprises like a flat tire, busted water pipe, huge electric bill, and obscene cell-phone charges. How we deal with new financial irritants determines if our Worry Circle is deluged or resilient.

Decisions get us into money problems, and different decisions can get us back out. Creditors aren't shy about changing their rules, which causes even more worries. It's easy to figure out if we're in a financial box. Having the courage to make a hard decision and repair a financial problem is tough—but it can be done.

Money is a finite commodity that poses infinite challenges. When we don't have *enough*, we think more money will solve our problems. When we get more, we realize that money doesn't eliminate our worries at all; sometimes money creates even more.

A friend of mine is the son of a billionaire and has been divorced six times; to me, too much money might sometimes be a bigger curse than having too little. All his wives, all his toys, all that money ... and he's still not happy. For him, money won't buy happiness, although I admit it does buy him access to nicer places to look for it.

When we live within our means, money's impact on our Worry Circle is minimized. Debt carries a heavy weight on our psyche, a load that burdens a feeling of obligation. Overextend, and anxiety compounds. Too much creates an emotional problem that causes many to lose sight of who they truly are. People suddenly career from being happy and well-balanced to depressed and out-of-balance.

Our fiscal lifeline is fixable. It may sometimes require recalibrating our lifestyle, but all hard choices take courage ... and discipline.

Until we are happy with who we are, we're never happy with what we have. Until we're grounded, *centered*, no amount of money is ever enough, since someone always has more.

I'm midway through my second million miles of flying around the world. The two countries I've visited that have the nicest and friendliest people are India and Cuba, none of whom worry about a 401-K. Money isn't what funds their kindness. Kindness is a gift to others and us. It's a better way of keeping score.

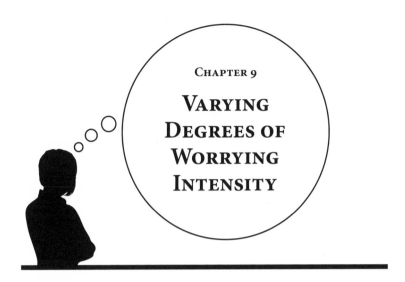

Worry spans a spectrum of emotions. Survival is at the top. Panic and adrenaline rushes come on suddenly. Road rage and air rage are eruptions at perceived violations of personal space. All of us feel varying degrees of emotional discomfort when our space is violated. Some people snap and turn violent.

Our "comfort zone" is our desired safety zone, which may expand or contract depending on the situation. In social interactions, Americans prefer an arm's length of space with someone they don't know; a stranger crowding us makes us uncomfortable. Conversely, in an intimate setting the comfort barrier is a foot or less.

When our desired space envelope is encroached upon, we instinctively react defensively. With road rage, a driver's space envelope feels invaded. We can't control a driver who is tailgating us. We *can* control our reaction. We can speed up, change lanes, slow down so they'll pass, pull over, or take an exit. And we can do all of this without unnecessary worry. We can choose not to react emotionally to the other person's disruptive behavior or outburst. Overriding our inborn, primal defense mechanism is a challenge, but knowing *why* someone in our rearview mirror upsets us gives us options. Park your worry, pick the best choice for the situation, act, then forget it.

Road rage is dangerous and such incidents will increase before they decrease. There are more cars on crowded roads, driven by an increasing number of stressed-out people, each jockeying for position.

Next time someone tailgates you, if you start to smolder, pull back. Resist the urge to battle. Responding inflames a situation. Be smart and back off.

The lens through which we look at life reflects the intensity and density of our Worry Circle. Our upbringing and life experiences impact how volatile our tolerance is. If raised in a family that fretted over nickels and dimes, we may, too. If our family was nomadic and moved a lot, we may uproot more often than people around us.

According to the United Nations, nearly 200 million people have immigrated to foreign countries, nearly all in search of life-improvement opportunities. These brave people leave the familiar by choice or by force for a number of reasons. Most typically: inadequate work opportunities, poor housing, excessive noise, unmanageable pollution, unsanitary conditions.

Immigrants must see daily life radically different than most Americans. What's stressful to them may not be stressful to us. Their space envelope may be significantly smaller than ours. Indians and Chinese live in societies with a billion people. They're used to crowds, being packed like sardines in trains and buses; U. S. midwest farmers aren't. Eastern Europeans live in apartments smaller than many American living rooms. Cramped living quarters are a non-issue to Eastern Europeans.

Maslow's Hierarchy of Needs

During World War II, psychologist Abraham Maslow wrote a paper titled "A Theory of Human Motivation." He detailed research identifying a five-step pyramid in a person's emotional fulfillment, finalized in "self-actualization." Maslow called this progressive behavioral journey a "Hierarchy of Needs."

The needs of the first stage must be met before we advance to the second, and so forth; the five steps are sequential. Step one is basic *survival* needs. From there, we progress toward the eventual end goal of personal fulfillment. Knowing this puts our Worry Circle issues into context, because worrying is normal.

What we worry about is okay, too. Using Maslow's five-step chart, we can understand *why* we worry about what we do.

Maslow's first stage identifies our basic physiological needs and biological requirements like food, water, oxygen, and thermal comfort. Second on the list are *safety* needs. Once our biological basics are met, security becomes important. In most parts of the United States, we take this for granted and seldom think about it—except if a negative situation is thrust upon us (e.g., Hurricane Katrina).

When we feel safe and secure, the next thing we pursue is *social acceptance.* We exchange love and affection to gain a sense of belonging.

After being socially accepted, fourth we pursue the need for *esteem*: self-esteem and the recognition of value from others. When we get it, we feel good. When we don't, we feel inferior and devalued. This step is at the core of the gang culture: If the members feel worthless, unimportant, and helpless to change anything, they react with violence.

The Worry Circle helps us at every step of Maslow's emotional dissection, but especially at the fourth step; because once we feel good and know how to sustain confident thoughts and feelings, we are free to pursue a higher purpose.

Maslow's fifth and final step, *self-actualization,* is our need to be and do what we were "born to do." To reach this stage in life, we must effectively manage our Worry Circle—free ourselves to pursue what matters most to us.

When we are hungry, scared, unsafe, unloved, ostracized, or lacking self-esteem, we are blocked from fulfilling our highest purpose. Because of that, we are unfulfilled. Managing our Worry Circle helps us to methodically proceed through each level of Maslow's pyramid until we finally earn the right to achieve a fulfilled life. To earn that right, we must free ourselves and pursue what matters most.

All six categories of things that typically fill our Worry Circle—individual, familial, social, environmental, work, and money—map directly to Maslow's hierarchy of needs. Regardless which of Maslow's five levels we're living at, when something we can control bugs us enough, we can take steps to resolve it. If we can't fix it, we kick it out. No room in our consciousness for doubt.

The further we are from basic survival needs, the more likely we can temper our worries. Perspective helps, as does the confidence that comes from knowing we can handle whatever shows up. Taking charge, and knowing when to let go, builds our courage. With courage comes belief in ourselves. When that happens, we have created a life full of purpose, meaning, and gratitude ... and we feel fulfilled. It's easier to be and stay happy, content with the life we've built. It's a safe haven, above where we used to be. As such, it's worth the hike to get there.

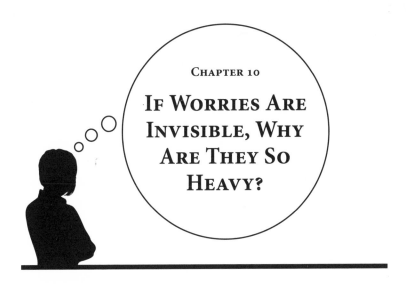

CHAPTER 10

IF WORRIES ARE INVISIBLE, WHY ARE THEY SO HEAVY?

When do people worry? Two things commonly start us worrying: accumulated thoughts and idle time. We worry more when alone than when preoccupied, in our spare time more than when busy. Loneliness and isolation foster worry problems because we have extra silent time to stew. People who are productive generally have fewer Worry Circle issues crowding their minds than people who aren't. Busy people are too preoccupied to daydream about a parenthetical thought concerning a hypothetical issue.

There is a massive difference, though, between a quiet person and a lonely one. By nature, people are gregarious animals. We live in groups and are friendly and sociable. So, if worry mounts, it's best not to withdraw. Instead, do the opposite. Reach out. Interface with others—especially positive people. It rubs off.

Worry eats up clock time—seconds, minutes, and hours—which is better served by being channeled into an area of personal investment. When the day is filled with passion, we don't dwell on worries (to the same extent as someone with nothing to do or no urgent higher purpose).

What we think shapes how we feel. How we feel triggers what we do (or don't do). Worries are conclusions we reach after processing a collected series of thoughts.

Behavior, therefore, results from action we take only after drawing an emotional conclusion. This conclusion results from on an emotional evaluation. From it, we decide that action is worth taking so we may (1) gain a positive reward, or (2) avoid a potential punishment. So, worry can be a prodding stimulus that inspires us to take action to make our life better (e.g., more education); or we can use it as a motivation to eradicate something negative (e.g., drop excess weight).

The clock time of our waking hours pass in one of four ways: it's spent, wasted, invested, or cherished. Worrying about things we cannot control is a *waste* of time. By refusing to worry about unnecessary things, we automatically waste less time. If we redirect those saved minutes into something we *cherish* (e.g., family), or *invest* them (e.g., personal or professional development), there's always a solid payback.

Excessive worry over an extended period takes a great toll, emotionally and physically. Managing our Worry Circle guards against long-term stress that may turn into listlessness, fatigue, physical decline, even mental or emotional instability. Health degradation doesn't affect just *us*. A downward spiral takes a negative toll on our family, friends, and associates.

Roughly speaking, one out of twenty people around the world deals with some form of depression. For some, the downward escalator carries them to the depths. However, when we consistently manage our worries *out* of our Worry Circle, we are proactively de-stressing and avoiding crumbling under the weight of all the harmful ways of thinking.

When we stay busy, we are helping to purify our Worry Circle, which frees us to focus on resolving our most important issues. Proactively resolving and retiring our Worry Circle issues gives us a strong sense of emotional accomplishment—which injects us with energy and inspiration. When an issue becomes important enough to solve (and the time arrives to deal with it), addressing it with determination builds confidence in us.

In business, we teach that there are three types of employees: those who make things happen, those who hope things will happen, and those who wonder what happened. Want to shed the burden of a troublesome issue? *Make* it happen.

Why Are We Happy, Why Are We Sad?

The mind is like a computer, so part of its functionality deals with calculations. We collect thoughts, either positive (+) or negative (-), from a myriad of stimuli, like advertisers. Commercial radio and television ads tell us what to think, how to feel, and what to do. Advertisers try to influence our behavior:

persuading us that we will benefit from their product, or that something undesirable will happen to us if we don't buy it. Fear sells more than inspiration; so more ads are negative than positive.

Opinions vary on how many ads the average person absorbs every day; the numbers range between 600 to more than 3,000. The industry consensus is that we see more advertisements in one year than fifty years ago people saw in a lifetime. So, the number of advertisements we'll be exposed to during our own lifetime ranges between eighteen to eighty *million*, based on an eighty-year lifespan. Internalizing bombardments like that explains why our head might feel a bit crowded. Our Worry Circle, too.

Advertisers should not have open access to our minds. So we should use our mind like a drawbridge: lower it when we want, raise it when we need to. Because what we think drives how we feel, we must police the thoughts that seek to enter our mind's castle. The goal is to collect more positive thoughts than negative ones. Do that, and we're happy. Flip-flop it—if the negatives outweigh the positives—and we're sad.

Disciplined Worry Circle management eliminates a huge source of negativity. By refusing to worry about what we can't control, we are raising our drawbridge against the relentless sources of negative invasions (which only eat at our energy and optimism). We also eliminate the wasted time and energy that go with intrusions.

We are happiest when centered, know how we got there,

and how to stay there. When balanced, it's easier to focus on the good in life and to be grateful for what we do have and not worry about what we don't have. When we have met the basic needs of Maslow's five-step life hierarchy, we can wake each day knowing we have enough. Life is charmed. We appreciate each day as an opportunity, and go to sleep feeling positive. Turn in at night positive, wake up positive. Go to sleep beaten, wake up negative. Sleep doesn't always reboot our outlook.

Sadness creeps in when we have too much idle time and dwell on what's wrong in our life instead of what's super about it. Life is a game. It has a beginning, middle, and end. As we play, we are forced to adjust to ever-changing rules. We play once, without practice or a dress rehearsal. As we play, no one, and no ad agency, has the right to cast dark clouds on our sunshine. Don't let others force those burdens on you.

We find in life what we look for. *Look for the good, see the good. Look for the bad, see the bad.* What we choose to look for is a personal choice, so it is totally "controllable." Happiness, therefore, is a choice. A superb and wonderful choice.

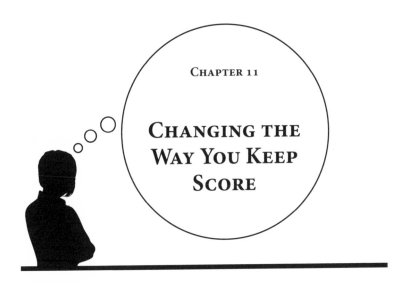

CHAPTER 11

CHANGING THE WAY YOU KEEP SCORE

Relax! You're winning!

Changing worry habits works best in tandem with changing how we judge our own success. During a robust economy, everybody makes money (or so it seems). But the score can change. Things are different now. When the ruler measures percentages of loss, rather than leapfrogs of gain, we must regain control of our mind space and think smarter.

When I was a younger man, I jogged to keep my weight down. Whenever I ran in a race, I judged success by minutes and seconds, fractions and splits. Each 5K, 10K, and 15K was me against the clock. In a marathon or half-marathon, it was me against the sundial. It was fun! The more I ran, the faster I got.

Two decades later, my knees started aching. Tendonitis got me, the bane of many a runner. No longer could I run as fast. When that happened, success changed. Success became measured by finishing safely.

Recently I had unexpected knee troubles. If everything goes right, a year after surgery I might be able to safely jog a slow and pain-free mile again. When I do, it will be an Olympic gold-medal moment. Success will be different now. As life evolves, so must how we keep score.

Tolerance Levels

Just as we have different personality types, we also have different thresholds of worry tolerance. People with a high threshold tend to downplay things, making anthills out of mountains. Others do the opposite; they hyperventilate at low-stress situations and make mountains out of anthills. Know yourself and know your worry tolerance. Learn to keep concerns in perspective. If you feel yourself losing perspective, tag a friend for help, an opinion, or support.

Worry Circle management does not measure success by perfection (nor does it mean putting pressure on others to be perfect). Perfect is too hard, too unrealistic. Just strive to be better, to have a happier life. Part of that is setting realistic goals. Are you getting better about being disciplined each day to better manage what you worry about? If your answer is yes, you're winning. If it's not (yet), keep at it. It's completely within your grasp.

How do we score Worry Circle success so that we are strengthening our self-image and self-esteem?

- *Money is not the scorecard.* Never has been. A car is not a scorecard; nor is the size of the home, the TV, the job title, the cubicle location, or brand of clothing. Worry Circle progress is powered by who we are, not what we have. This bears repeating: *Until we're happy with who we are, we'll never be happy with what we have.* It's true for all of us, every day. Material things come and go. The true score when measuring Worry Circle effectiveness is how good we feel between head and heart. When those two are in balance, we are winning the game.

- *Stigmas, embarrassment, and courage.* All of us have things in life we'd like to do over—so let go of past frailties. No baggage in the Worry Circle. Drop it. Leave it behind. Move on. We must let go of our rainy yesterdays to find our bright and sunny todays and tomorrows.

- *Ownership.* Do you own issues or whine about them? Do you face challenges that come your way or complain about being a victim because circumstances are unfair? Ownership is a box on the scorecard. Make sure you can check it off. Victimization does not exist.

- *Don't be too hard on yourself.* Changing habitual ways of thinking and reacting takes effort and repetition. It's not instant. So, in the next chapter, we cover the seven cardinal rules of managing the Worry Circle. In the last chapter is an exercise to define exactly what you aspire to be. Commit to learning to master these things, and celebrate improvement. Every progressive step matters. Each brings us closer to living with joy and a full and peaceful heart.

Process-driven, disciplined thinking—and reacting—can be a lot of fun. We learn to leave behind the burdens of our cluttered, disorganized mind. We confront our Worry Circle issues (large and small) and handle them with confidence. It's a beautiful way to live.

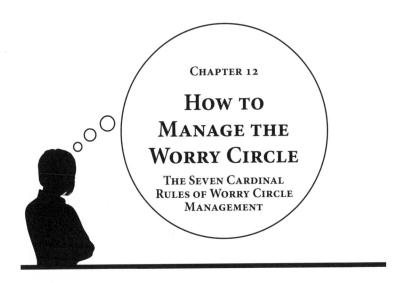

CHAPTER 12

How to Manage the Worry Circle

The Seven Cardinal Rules of Worry Circle Management

Worry Circle management is a systematic policing of our mind to block out unsolvable concerns. It's not some gimmick that promises to abolish worry. Human nature says we're going to worry. Trust me: No matter how good we get at Worry Circle management, we'll still worry. What changes is how much better we handle it.

The seven cardinal rules of managing the Worry Circle provide a simple, orderly, and reliable *process* for culling out bad worries so we can focus on owning issues we *can* control to keep our life in better balance.

Why must we manage the Worry Circle? If we don't, it's difficult (if not impossible) to remain balanced, positive, and in control of our emotions during a trying or stressful time. If we have no strategy and must deal with everything life dishes out (in its unfiltered, haphazard stream), we are forced into an endless chain of knee-jerk reactions trying to fix things we have no possible hope of fixing. Faced with a relentless mess, our ability to remain in consistent control of our emotions is virtually nil.

What enables rock solid Worry Circle management? All seven rules are important. The first is pretty obvious.

1. *You've got to drink the Kool-Aid.* The fundamental base of managing our worries requires a commitment to own what we *choose* to worry about ... and kick out the rest. Own the worries you can control. Compartmentalize the worries you can influence into two smaller boxes: (1) a segment you can control and own, and (2) the rest of the things that are uncontrollable (and immediately get rid of them). Worries about totally uncontrollable things are poison. Don't allow them between the ears.

2. *Balance all three of your heads.* Every person has three heads, not one. The first is preoccupied with how we want to appear to others. The second is worried about how we *are* perceived by others. The third doesn't care about the other two; it only cares about who we really are—which is where our power rests. People unable to control their Worry Circle aren't balancing the conflicts and collisions between their three heads. Since Worry Circle strength comes from the inside out, we must be comfortable with our third head (who we really are). Then we can balance the other two.

3. *We find in life what we look for.* One of my favorite

stories is "Gretchen and the Shark's Teeth," a recitation of how one of life's most valuable lessons was taught to me by a pint-sized four-year-old. I was in college at the time and forced to babysit due to a freakish alignment of the zodiac. I was scared. I wasn't a babysitter. I was a college kid.

To kill time, I drove us fifteen miles from my campus in Jacksonville, Florida to the beach at Mayport. My plan was to beachcomb, using the kid as slave labor. A dredging ship was anchored offshore, pumping a steady flow of fresh sand back up onto the beach to rebuild what erosion had washed out. A lot of shark's teeth came tumbling out with the sand and glistened in the sun. The pickings were easy.

At the end of our walk, I had a handful of small shiny ebony triangles. I turned to Gretchen, who was five paces away. Her tiny hand clutched a white Styrofoam cup filled to the brim with giant teeth. Her smallest was twice the size of my largest. I was incredulous. I had found three times as many but none were as large as hers. There had to be a reason and I wanted to learn it.

"Gretchen," I asked sweetly, "why are all of yours so big?"

She looked up at me with certainty. "'Cause that's what I was looking for."

I nearly fell down at her simplicity, and I never forgot this valuable life lesson: We find in life what we look for.

When we look for good, that's what we find. Look for bad and *that's* what we find. Worry Circle management kicks the appropriate negative influences out of our mind, so we can focus on the positive.

4. *The list of things we do not do*. Everyone has a mental list of things we don't do: like robbing banks, being mean to kids, poisoning dogs, taking heroin, stealing, or stiffing efficient waitstaff in restaurants. Our list reflects our core values and beliefs, and sets the behavioral boundaries of our lives. Worry Circle management treats things we can't control with the same grave importance as these other bad things. Worrying about things we can't control is toxic. We don't do it. We do not drink emotional poison.

5. *The list of things we used to do but don't do any more!* Our behaviors evolve. Just like we have a mental list of Things We Do Not Do, we also have a list of Things We Used to Do But Don't Do Any More. For example, many people used to smoke but quit, used to drink and drive but don't now, used to eat at McDonald's but stopped after seeing Morgan Spurlock's movie, *SuperSize Me*. Millions of Americans do not shop at Walmart, believing the mega-giant's predatory pricing strategies do more harm than good for small communities. From a Worry Circle perspective, add to this list worrying about things you cannot control. It's something you used to do, but refuse to do any more.

6. *Living with passion and urgency.* Goals cure boredom. When we wake up energized about life and the balance we've worked hard to attain, getting things done comes easily. When we stay busy, we have less time to worry. Passion and energy fuel achievement. So to manage our Worry Circle, we live each day with a strong and prideful sense of purpose. There is an adage in business that says, "If you want something done, give it to a busy person." You want to be that busy person.

7. *Staying true to your Daily Dozen.* The Daily Dozen is our personalized list that precisely defines who we aspire to be. You will craft yours in chapter fourteen. The truer we stay to our Daily Dozen list, the fewer emotional conflicts we have. All twelve of these handpicked traits are core to our being and each one we are empowered to pursue.

There is a strong relationship between what gets housed in our Worry Circle and the list of our Daily Dozen. Controllable worry issues that relate to the core values of our Daily Dozen are prioritized. What is not relevant to our Daily Dozen is secondary. Uncontrollable concerns are kicked out. The Daily Dozen helps us rank, in order of importance, what matters to us most.

These seven rules help us control how we handle life's agitations. When we embrace all seven, managing our Worry Circle becomes easy. It's a process that is replicable even in a time of high stress, enabling us to be strong from the inside out. Embrace these rules and they'll never let you down.

Is Life in Balance?

PERSONAL   **BEHAVIORAL**

OUR CONSCIENCE

Who we are.   **What we do.**
(defines self -image)   (fuels self-esteem)

Are our three heads   Are our three
of the "three-headed   heads reconciled
person" reconciled?   behaviorally? Do
How we want to   our deeds match our
appear to others,   intentions? Are our
how we do appear   behaviors consistent
to others, and who   with our Daily Dozen
we really are. Are   … even when no one
we happy, content,   is watching?
and fulfilled? Are
we in control of our
worries, or are our
worries controlling
us?

How do we attain balance and inner peace? How can we be happier?

The Dalai Lama has a talent for saying a lot while saying very little. During an interview, he was asked the secret of happiness.

"Do more, want less," he answered.

He suggests that if we do more for others and want less for ourselves, we will create a happier state of mind. When our life has progressed upward through Maslow's first four levels of basic needs, we have plenty. How well balanced and happy we are after that is up to us.

How do we get over the burdens and regrets of the past?

Do four things: (1) Own that it's time to eradicate what worries us. (2) Eliminate all venomous attitudes. (3) Change our point of view. Study both sides of the lens, especially when dealing with matters of the heart. Not every issue requires a right and wrong. Sometimes differences just "are." (4) Forgive. Forgive others and forgive ourselves. Forgiving is part of the new way we choose to keep score.

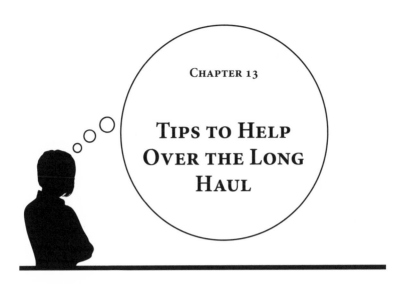

CHAPTER 13

TIPS TO HELP OVER THE LONG HAUL

This series of tips will help you stay in command of your Worry Circle, day after day, year after year. They are grouped into three coaching levels.

Major Reminders

These are four very important considerations to assist with sustained success.

When Facing a Lifestyle Change

Some worries are created by choices we are forced to make when pondering whether to make a major change in our status quo. Among the biggies: getting married, moving, downsizing, taking a new job with a new company, borrowing a large sum of money, or splurging on an expensive vacation.

Before the plunge, take the time to measure the impact these changes might have on your tolerance for worry. I thought I could handle the stress of getting married. On the way to the church in Baltimore, I had the driver pull over where I got sick at the side of the road. Nerves trumped my then-fledgling Worry Circle management skills. Proof that for some it's helpful to embrace and absorb the impact of big decisions out over time.

Go Outside Your Normal Comfort Zone

Accept your true feelings. Do NOT ignore how you feel about something that's causing you an unfamiliar amount of emotional distress. If you sense that what you're dealing with is beyond your comfort zone, seek unbiased, professional help or the private counsel of a trusted confidant. Worry Circle management helps us decide what to own between our ears (and what to get rid of). However, there are times where other viewpoints are better than one.

Give Yourself Room to Rebound

If you've been forced to deal with a significant, negative emotional experience, give yourself time to reflect and recover. Years ago, I made a big mistake and tried to teach an important week-long pilot class two days after burying my father. I had no business being in front of the room. I was there physically but a million miles from Mars emotionally. The first day was a career-threatening disaster. A friend of mine volunteered to tag in to save me and protect the integrity of the program. I took the week off and needed every second of it.

Work to Live, Rather Than Live to Work

The more submerged we get into a one-dimension existence

that hinges on business, the more likely we are to be impacted by changes beyond our control, things like: increased competition, economic downturns, uncontrollable attacks, and unexpected survival restructuring. An enormous burden of stress is tied to job security, an increased workload, a mismatched skill set, impossible deadlines, political backstabbing, and dead-end careers. As our thoughts become polluted, so do our perceptions. "Secret agendas" appear from the vapors. We see what's broken instead of what's good. We dig in to argue, rather than build on whatever we have in common. When overtime replaces leisure time, family problems and money arguments soon follow.

Five Other Tips that Help Over Time
Manage Your Time Smartly

The world is full of busy people yet short of productive ones. The pressure to achieve is great. Time is finite. If you feel like you're spinning and not getting the traction you want out of life, stop and analyze the productivity of your days.

Waking hours are occupied in one of four ways: time is wasted, spent, invested, or cherished. To gain a better quality of life, study your daily time choices. How many waking hours fall into each category? A fulfilling life maximizes our time. To do that, we need to cherish and invest as much time as we possibly can, and decrease the amount of time we waste or spend on low-value activities.

Time choices we can control. Worrying about things we can't control is a waste of time, so when we stop worrying about them we can re-channel that time into investment or cherish time.

Frustration is the residue of lost opportunity and with frustration comes Worry Circle angst. By eliminating poor time-use choices, we can maximize opportunities and eradicate Worry Circle issues. The more time we cherish and invest, the less time remains to waste. Smart choices are key. The place to start is banning uncontrollable concerns from the Worry Circle and focusing solely on doing things that matter most to you.

Call Time Out When in Overload

When you've entered a period of increased worry and your mind is more crowded than usual, force yourself to take a minimum of three breaks each day to reenergize. Build them into your schedule ... and take them. During these timeouts, focus only on positive resolutions. Double-check what's inside your Worry Circle, toss out anything that doesn't belong there, and recommit to managing the remaining controllable anxieties. Draw strength from previous successes.

Protect Your Mind Space

What we feed our mind, our body wants. Be a disciplined gatekeeper of your thoughts. Maximize positive emotional experiences to minimize negative ones. Doing so is a personal choice. Remember that TV and radio ads bombard us, and half of what's scripted urges messages of negative consequence. So, don't let others decide what's good for you. Guard yourself. Monitor what you allow into your mind. One way to minimize the noise is to turn it off.

Avoid the Reflexive Loop

The reflexive loop is a series of predictable, repetitive habits. Some people live in a reflexive loop, others don't. The broader our range of experiences, the less time we spend in the reflexive loop. We think in new and fresher ways, so our emotional reaction when something disrupts our status quo is less intense. To minimize the trap of the reflexive loop, try new things. Be open to change. We grow old in a hurry when trapped in the reflexive loop: behaving robotically, change-averse, common destinations, park in the same place, eat the same thing every day. Don't do that. Experiment. Go new places, try new things. Make a game out of mixing things up.

Write Down What You Want to Accomplish

Write down your short-term, mid-term, and longer-term goals, what you'd like to accomplish. Then prioritize. Short-term is within one year, mid-term is one to three years, longer term over three years. Keep these lists handy. Refer to them often and they'll become part of you. You'll *want* to achieve them. Hopefully the words "Manage the Worry Circle" are at the top of every list.

Super Tips to Use As Needed

Stay Confident

When your behaviors can remedy a situation, draw strength from that self-assurance. If an issue is bugging you, deal with it it. Step up. Action makes us stronger. Action lessens our emotional vulnerability.

If You're Slipping Into a Funk ...

Improve your fitness. Good things grow from feeling better.

Make Sound Nutritional Choices

The worse shape we're in, the more our self-esteem takes a hit. Be in tune with what you're eating and drinking. What digests easily and provides energy? What does your system struggle with? Ingested choices directly impact how we feel physically. Mentally, too.

Don't Take Yourself Too Seriously

No matter how frustrating things might be for us, billions of other people on the planet don't care. So, don't unnecessarily burden yourself. Impatience and intensity are bigger curses than virtues, and trying to do too much, too fast, causes frustration and stress. Take life in stride. "Chill out," as they say.

Demonstrate Compassion

Personal success isn't the same as it is for someone else. We are our own measure. A full life is to relentlessly challenge yourself—from a thousand different angles—while rooting for others and cheering them on. Be happy for others' success. When they are struggling, help them. Caring is free. Become great at it. It boosts self-esteem.

Know Yourself

It's important to like who you are. Staying centered comes from inside. It's your head and heart in balance. When you feel good about who you are, everything is easier.

Be Flexible

Times change. We must, too. The easier we embrace

change, the less we worry about it. (*Reminder:* Smart change management is in chapter two.)

Judge Less, Seek to Understand More

We are all raised in different experiences, so we usually see situations differently than others. This is okay. This is normal. This is being human. Rather than dwell on differences, celebrate others to be the way they are.

Cultivate a Like-minded Circle of Friends

Minimize time with negative people. Hang out with positive, upbeat ones. Who you interface with (or don't) is a choice. Listening to negative people brings us down. Positive people energize and inspire us.

Look Out for Number One—Yourself!

If something's preventing you from having a happy, healthy lifestyle, don't keep ducking it. Fix it. Tomorrow is always the busiest day of the year, because that's when people plan on doing things. Why wait? If you need to change something, start now.

Don't Worry How Others Keep Score

We judge ourselves by our intentions. Others judge us by our actions and achievements. So what? Don't fret about what others think. Know yourself. If you're comfortable in your own skin, and live and behave by good intentions, good things will result. The scorecard that matters isn't someone else's. It's yours.

Smile More!

Be a smiling machine! Smiling is infectious. The more you do it, the easier it gets.

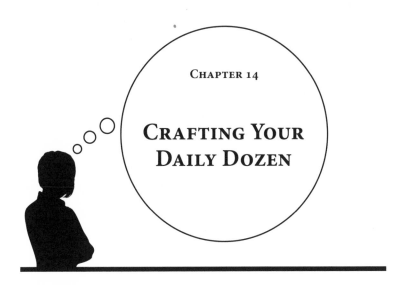

CHAPTER 14

CRAFTING YOUR DAILY DOZEN

This exercise helps you define who you aspire to be (not who you are today). The more time you invest in this exercise, the more you'll get out of it. The directions are simple and straightforward, but the exercise takes a good deal of introspection to maximize its utility.

Brainstorm twelve *personal* traits that are very important to you. These are things you want to see in yourself, so take plenty of time to think this through. When you've finished your list, resume reading.

-
-
-

-
-
-
-
-
-
-
-
-

Now study what you've come up with. Then go back through the twelve items and number the bullets in their order of importance to you. Identify the most important and work your way down through to whatever ranks twelfth.

Once the traits are ranked in the proper order, reread each one. Can it be more accurately explained, clearer, more precise? Each item's phraseology should exactly describe the point.

After you perfect all twelve items, type the list and print it. Scissor the list and post it where you'll see it all the time, in plain sight. Even better, print extras. Post them wherever you're likely to see them. This is your Daily Dozen—who you aspire to be.

I wrote mine two decades ago while sitting on a seawall in Bimini, Bahamas. I wasn't happy at the time and knew I needed to decide who I truly wanted to be. For many men, this silent soul-search is a rite of adult passage. We may always be our father's sons, but there is a step beyond that: becoming our own man.

I sat on that seawall for three hours, through a tide change, identifying twelve qualities about the person I wanted to be that felt vital to my future happiness. The hardest part was having every word serve a purpose, to capture precisely what I was feeling.

When I returned home to Miami, I typed and laminated the list and glued it to a magnet at the side of the filing cabinet near where I write. It's small but mighty. Here it is:

TED'S DAILY DOZEN

1. Be a better husband.

2. Be a better father.

3. Perform a quality day of work.

4. Eat sensibly.

5. Avoid alcohol.

6. Exercise.

7. Support my wife's personal growth.

8. Stay positive.

9. Be nice.

10. Make a stranger laugh.

11. Pursue own personal growth.

12. Write something.

Number one, if I'm a great spouse, it's hard to be a lousy parent. My wife is an angel of patience and kindness, a Type B reserved personality. "Saint Bonnie" the family calls her. As with any long-term relationship, we've had our ups and downs. But when I'm the cause of a "down," I look over my Daily Dozen and my personal shortfall glares back at me like a laser beam, which instantly reminds me of my core values. I then know what I need to repair. This tool prevents me from ducking ownership of what matters most to me. Having this list in plain view forces me to manage my Worry Circle immediately.

Number two on my list is solved by honoring number one. Number three: I sleep better after a day of good work than a wasted day of putzing around. Marvin Fisher, a grocery store meatcutter who dropped out of high school, taught me the value of hard work. He was my boss when I was working my way through college. He wasn't an educated man, but Marvin was a remarkable worker. I had to bust my tail to stay anywhere close to his output. Every day Marvin showed up ready to work, and every day he dared the rest of us to keep up. His sustaining work ethic overpowered his lack of education. Never once did Marvin Fisher back into the pay window. By example, he taught me a powerful life lesson: Work is not an entitlement. It's a privilege. We're all given the same amount of time, so our reputation is gained by what we accomplish, not by what we promise.

Number four: Eating sensibly. Straightforward enough, complicated only by red licorice Twizzlers and my fresh-baked nemesis: chocolate éclairs.

Number five is because of my late mother. The bottle beat her at fifty-three. None of the four of her children—my brother, two sisters, and me—will ever travel that road. Demons are formidable foes, and not everyone can beat them. Having watched what happens when someone loses, the four of us decided to never underestimate the opposition.

Number six: Exercise releases endorphins and they make me feel better. What I'm capable of these days isn't close to my younger days, but the value of a good workout remains remarkable. There's no better opportunity to clear my head by thinking through what matters while toning my body. Head benefits. Heart benefits. One of the best free things a person can ever do.

Number seven: My lovely wife is a giver, not a taker, generous to a fault, so she's always fun to root for, especially when she's involved with something that matters to her. Because of that, supporting her personal growth is important to me.

Numbers eight and nine: A pair of interpersonal skills: stay positive and be nice. I learned these from two guys who impacted my life in good ways at different times. George Simmons mentored me in the late 1980s when I was teaching at the Xerox International Center for Training and Management Development in Leesburg, Virginia. Every day he bugged me to stay positive. George lived that way—until he died on September 11, 2001, when he and his wife were on the plane that was skyjacked into the Pentagon.

Being nice as a life lesson came from an unlikely source.

One weekday afternoon in the summer of 1990, Hall of Fame boxing trainer Angelo Dundee spent two hours with me in his Pembroke Pines, Florida office. He made a point of explaining to me the importance of being nice. Angelo is a terrific, charismatic, and *nice* man, and he is much beloved in a tough and shady business.

A few years later, Angelo mailed me a reminder card: "Keep being nice!" Several years later he sent me another that made me laugh: "Keep slipping punches." Timeless reminders, especially now that the economy is wobbling like a bicycle with two bent wheels. Angie's first note is a reminder. The second one is his boxing terminology for the best way to deal with Worry Circle issues. Magnets hold both cards side by side on my file cabinet, a foot from my Daily Dozen list.

Being nice is free. Staying balanced and managing our Worry Circle helps us slip punches that otherwise might tag us on the chin.

Numbers ten, eleven, and twelve: Laughter, personal growth, and writing are core elements of what makes me happy personally. Laughter is orange juice for my soul. I love comedy and the sound of spontaneous laughter. Love to write it, watch it, and applaud it.

To push my personal growth, I remember a quote from Muhammad Ali, the legendary three-time heavyweight boxing champion whom Angelo trained. Long after retiring, the champ was asked if he missed being the flamboyant world figure of his twenties.

"A man who looks at life at fifty, " he replied, "the same he did at twenty has wasted thirty years."

Pretty simple. Keep moving. Never quit growing.

I write something every day. Writing is a craft. It takes a ton of work but I love the work. When I miss a day I feel like I cheated myself out of something valuable, like I shortchanged myself out of creating something worthwhile. To writers, a piece of paper is nothing until they write on it. What it is after that is up to them.

Creating our Daily Dozen list is the first step to living it. Mine carries me past uncertainties and leads me directly to the man I still want to be.

We are always growing. It never stops. A life well-lived is a relentless pursuit to become better at things that matter to us.

Living in steadfast pursuit of who we aspire to be—Maslow's fifth and highest level of self-actualization—is half the work. The other half is managing our Worry Circle so that we can progress along the way.

It's a pretty good feeling to look in the mirror and like who you see. All it takes is a splash of heart and a dash of commitment. Once those two are mixed together, positive change is never as hard as it seems. Best of all, we find the biggest shark's tooth of all: the life we're looking for. And what could be better than that?

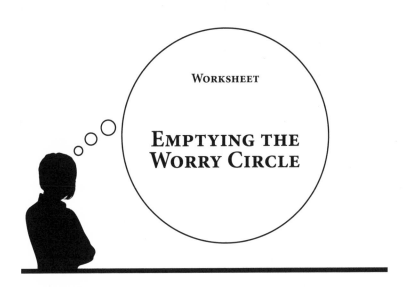

WORKSHEET

EMPTYING THE WORRY CIRCLE

The following worksheet is meant to help you manage your worries. Extras are provided. Fill one out and post it in highly visible areas around your home and office as a reminder.

EMPTYING THE WORRY CIRCLE

(For each identified worry, check only one of these three columns.)

CATEGORY & WORRY	Can you control it?	Can you influence it but not resolve it?	Is this totally beyond your control?
Personal Worries			
Familial Worries			
Social Worries			
Environmental Worries			
Work-related Worries			
Money worries			
Summary:	Embrace these.	Compartmentalize these. Own what you can control. Jettison the rest.	Block these out of your mind. They're not allowed in.

EMPTYING THE WORRY CIRCLE

(For each identified worry, check only one of these three columns.)

CATEGORY & WORRY	Can you control it?	Can you influence it but not resolve it?	Is this totally beyond your control?
Personal Worries			
Familial Worries			
Social Worries			
Environmental Worries			
Work-related Worries			
Money worries			
Summary:	Embrace these.	Compartmentalize these. Own what you can control. Jettison the rest.	Block these out of your mind. They're not allowed in.

EMPTYING THE WORRY CIRCLE

(For each identified worry, check only one of these three columns.)

CATEGORY & WORRY	Can you control it?	Can you influence it but not resolve it?	Is this totally beyond your control?
Personal Worries			
Familial Worries			
Social Worries			
Environmental Worries			
Work-related Worries			
Money worries			
Summary:	Embrace these.	Compartmentalize these. Own what you can control. Jettison the rest.	Block these out of your mind. They're not allowed in.

EMPTYING THE WORRY CIRCLE

(For each identified worry, check only one of these three columns.)

CATEGORY & WORRY	Can you control it?	Can you influence it but not resolve it?	Is this totally beyond your control?
Personal Worries			
Familial Worries			
Social Worries			
Environmental Worries			
Work-related Worries			
Money worries			
Summary:	Embrace these.	Compart-mentalize these. Own what you can control. Jettison the rest.	Block these out of your mind. They're not allowed in.

EMPTYING THE WORRY CIRCLE

(For each identified worry, check only one of these three columns.)

CATEGORY & WORRY	Can you control it?	Can you influence it but not resolve it?	Is this totally beyond your control?
Personal Worries			
Familial Worries			
Social Worries			
Environmental Worries			
Work-related Worries			
Money worries			
Summary:	Embrace these.	Compartmentalize these. Own what you can control. Jettison the rest.	Block these out of your mind. They're not allowed in.

Other books by Ocean Palmer

TUKI BANJO, SUPERSTAR

THE RISE AND FALL OF PIGGY CHURCH

MAXIMUM HORSEPOWER

HIGHWAY TO SOMEWHERE

JURASSIC TROUT*

SEARCHING FOR TENDULKAR*

12 MILES TO PARADISE*

RICH WITHOUT MONEY*

CRITTERS, FISH & OTHER TROUBLEMAKERS*

*as Ted Simendinger